KU-411-444

Establishing a Culture
of Patient Safety

This book is due for return on or before the last date shown below.

28/08/23		

Also available from ASQ Quality Press:

Communication: The Key to Effective Leadership
Judith Ann Pauley and Joseph F. Pauley

*Using ISO 9001 in Healthcare: Applications for Quality Systems,
Performance Improvement, Clinical Integration, and Accreditation*
James M. Levett, MD and Robert G. Burney, MD

*Lean Doctors: A Bold and Practical Guide to Using Lean Principles to
Transform Healthcare Systems, One Doctor at a Time*
Aneesh Suneja with Carolyn Suneja

Quality Function Deployment and Lean Six Sigma Applications in Public Health
Grace L. Duffy, John W. Moran, and William Riley

The Public Health Quality Improvement Handbook
Ron Bialek, John W. Moran, and Grace L. Duffy

*Root Cause Analysis and Improvement in the Healthcare Sector:
A Step-by-Step Guide*
Bjørn Andersen, Tom Fagerhaug, and Marti Beltz

*Solutions to the Healthcare Quality Crisis: Cases and Examples of Lean
Six Sigma in Healthcare*
Soren Bisgaard, editor

On Becoming Exceptional: SSM Health Care's Journey to Baldrige and Beyond
Sister Mary Jean Ryan, FSM

Journey to Excellence: Baldrige Health Care Leaders Speak Out
Kathleen Goonan, editor

*A Lean Guide to Transforming Healthcare: How to Implement Lean Principles
in Hospitals, Medical Offices, Clinics, and Other Healthcare Organizations*
Thomas G. Zidel

*Benchmarking for Hospitals: Achieving Best-in-Class Performance without
Having to Reinvent the Wheel*
Victor Sower, Jo Ann Duffy, and Gerald Kohers

*Lean-Six Sigma for Healthcare, Second Edition: A Senior Leader Guide to
Improving Cost and Throughput*
Greg Butler, Chip Caldwell, and Nancy Poston

Lean Six Sigma for the Healthcare Practice: A Pocket Guide
Roderick A. Munro

To request a complimentary catalog of ASQ Quality Press publications, call
800-248-1946, or visit our website at http://www.asq.org/quality-press.

Establishing a Culture of Patient Safety

Improving Communication, Building Relationships, and Using Quality Tools

Judith Ann Pauley and Joseph F. Pauley

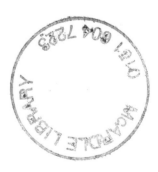

ASQ Quality Press
Milwaukee, Wisconsin

American Society for Quality, Quality Press, Milwaukee 53203
Printed in the United States of America
16 15 14 13 12   5 4 3 2

Library of Congress Cataloging-in-Publication Data

Pauley, Judith A.
  Establishing a culture of patient safety : improving communication, building
relationships, and using quality tools / Judith Ann Pauley and Joseph F. Pauley.
      p. cm.
  Includes bibliographical references and index.
  ISBN 978-0-87389-819-5 (alk. paper)
  1. Hospitals—Administration. 2. Medical errors—Prevention. 3. Communication
in medicine. 4. Physician and patient. 5. Medical care—Safety measures. I. Pauley,
Joseph F. II. Title.
  [DNLM: 1. Hospital Administration. 2. Medical Errors—prevention & control.
3. Comprehensive Health Care—methods. 4. Models, Organizational. 5. Professional-
Patient Relations. 6. Safety Management. WX 153]

  RA971.P38 2011
  362.11068—dc23

                                                                    2011017946

Publisher: William A. Tony
Acquisitions Editor: Matt Meinholz
Project Editor: Paul O'Mara
Production Administrator: Randall Benson

ASQ Mission: The American Society for Quality advances individual, organizational, and community excellence worldwide through learning, quality improvement, and knowledge exchange.

Attention Bookstores, Wholesalers, Schools, and Corporations: ASQ Quality Press
books, video, audio, and software are available at quantity discounts with bulk
purchases for business, educational, or instructional use. For information, please
contact ASQ Quality Press at 800-248-1946, or write to ASQ Quality Press,
P.O. Box 3005, Milwaukee, WI 53201-3005.

To place orders or to request a free copy of the ASQ Quality Press Publications
Catalog, visit our website at http://www.asq.org/quality-press.

 Printed on acid-free paper

Quality Press
600 N. Plankinton Ave.
Milwaukee, WI 53203-2914
E-mail: authors@asq.org

The Global Voice of Quality™

To

Major General (ret.) Gale S. Pollock, former Acting
Surgeon General of the United States Army, for her
friendship, for sharing her leadership skills with us,
and for recognizing how the concepts of Process
Communication can improve the healthcare provided to
the army heroes wounded in battle defending our country
and to their family members who have remained behind.

And to

Dr. Taibi Kahler, the clinical psychologist who made
the discoveries on which the concepts of Process
Communication are based, for his genius, for his
friendship, and for improving our lives and the lives
of all those we come in contact with every day.

And especially to

All the healthcare professionals who provide
outstanding medical care to millions of patients every
year, especially those who have dealt patiently with
our idiosyncrasies and provided excellent medical
care and advice to us throughout our lives.

Contents

List of Figures and Tables

Foreword

Human interaction can be complicated. It probably always has been. Even in the days when communities of our ancestors huddled together in caves for protection and for warmth, living together in proximity for extended periods, it was the same. As they negotiated or resolved to establish an agreed pecking order, and as they rationed out their (often scarce) resources, their skills in being able to relate effectively and constructively to one another were tested—and, indeed, the very survival of their community often depended on it. Not to mention the challenges of keeping their youngest ones safe, dealing with their impulsive and rebellious teenagers, and caring for their sick and elderly. All this required sophisticated social interaction. One would have to think that nothing has changed.

Well, almost nothing. The same bases for these intricacies of human behaviour remain. But what is different now is the environment in which they play out: It is much more complex and demanding. It places much greater stress on its inhabitants. The senses are bombarded with a greater range of stimuli that require rapid and specific responses. So in many ways, the range of skills required for effective daily functioning has become significantly more complex. It is not so much that the technology we use (whether it be cars or computers) has become more complicated, but more that the array of systems and processes with which we now have to comply has become increasingly complicated. Nowhere is this more evident than in the area of health services.

That is where this book comes in. It is true that the technology and techniques of medicine are advancing rapidly, concomitant with an ever-expanding knowledge base, and that this necessitates high levels of cognitive and technical expertise by those who provide medical care. Yet, this is not where the real challenge lies. Rather, it is that these advances also demand that all healthcare workers communicate effectively and work collaboratively, an absolute necessity if the complex processes that have been built up around healthcare provision are to function properly.

Why have these processes around the delivery of healthcare become so complex? Not surprisingly, there are several reasons. One obvious one is the explosion in knowledge and skills required within each specialty area. This has led to an increased level of specialization and delineation of the roles and responsibilities of each member of the workforce. In turn, this means that, more than ever before, health workers are dependent on those around them for support if they are to perform their work correctly.

But there is another reason, one that relates to patient safety. The public now expects good outcomes to be routine. Previously, complications were assumed mainly to be related to patient factors (e.g., old age, poor healing, comorbidity, or the patient not following the doctor's instructions correctly) or to limitations in available technology. It was assumed that medical staff, being honest and having integrity, were infrequent contributors to poor outcomes. Now—and this book highlights the importance of this aspect—we realize that many, if not most, unexpected adverse events are due to human factors, specifically the actions and behaviour of those looking after the patients.

In short, medical error leads to adverse events, and adverse events lead to poor clinical outcomes. Understanding how medical error occurs is the first stage in reducing its incidence. This book reviews the evidence that certain types of human behaviour contribute to errors occurring. Moreover, it also shows the degree to which these types of behaviour are predictable. Fortunately, they can be recognized and dealt with, not only by health professionals reflecting on themselves but also by colleagues. Understanding the role of personality types and recognizing the effects of stress and distress allow a greater degree of collegiality and a more collaborative and supportive environment. The authors outline the tools available to achieve this. Put simply, once we have the tools that have been shown to improve behaviour (or eliminate those behaviours that contribute to mistakes), we will be on the road to providing a safer health system.

This book is a welcome addition to our libraries, as it applies the Process Communication Model® to the health sector. We already know that human factors—primarily behaviour affected by varying degrees of stress—contribute to medical errors. Here we have a tome that reminds us that perhaps the most productive way to minimize medical error is to study how well-intentioned and committed health specialists function and communicate. Additionally, it encourages us to adopt some very specific tools to influence this behaviour in a way that eliminates many of the human factors that contribute to the high incidence of medical error that plagues our health services.

Spencer W. Beasley, MB, ChB (Otago),
MS (Melbourne), F.R.A.C.S.
Professor of Paediatric Surgery, Christchurch School of
Medicine and Health Sciences, University of Otago
Former Chair of the Board of Surgical Education and
Training, Royal Australasian College of Surgeons

The healthcare industry today faces many challenges. In spite of the fact that technology has enabled healthcare professionals to provide the highest quality of healthcare in history, raise the life expectancy of our population, and find cures for illness after illness, we still are challenged to improve patient safety and patient satisfaction. Our challenge is daunting: improve the quality of healthcare, and improve patient safety to a "perfect" level in a labor-intensive business model that will remain labor intensive and people dependent for the foreseeable future. This people-dependent business must ensure that employee engagement and satisfaction are also a constant focus. To accomplish these tasks, it is essential to improve communication among all members of the healthcare team (doctors, nurses, administrators, and patients) and to reduce their distress levels.

When working daily in situations dealing with patients who have suffered life-threatening heart attacks or strokes or who have been in accidents, stress is inevitable. The key is to be able to deal with stress in positive ways, thereby turning it into positive stress rather than negative stress (distress). This book provides a tool that can be applied to accomplish these goals.

In an effort to improve communication and reduce the distress in our hospital, the leadership was trained in the concepts of Process Communication. It worked. Tools that could be applied were applied. Leaders who struggled with one another and with certain relationships suddenly had a different lens to view not only their statements but also the reception of their statements. Listening improved. And we saw results. We saw improvement in employee engagement. These concepts enhanced our ability to deal positively with individual issues as well as hospital-wide management issues. This resulted in a 6% improvement in employee engagement in one year (2009) and has enabled us to move the entire organization to the next level.

I learned a lot about myself and about communication gaps that I unintentionally allowed; but, for the first time, I have a tool that I can use with my children, their teachers, my wife, my staff, patients in the hospital, and everyone with whom I interact. The concepts have enabled me to be a better manager because I now listen for clues to indicate how to interact successfully with the person in front of me at any given moment. In addition, senior leaders in the hospital now individualize the way they communicate with their employees on the issues facing them. They are able to respond to each person in the way that makes the most sense to each individual.

For example, those who perceive the world through their emotions want to know that their bosses care about them and are willing to listen to them and allow them to discuss their feelings. Those who perceive the world through thoughts don't care about that. They come to meetings with their list of things they want to discuss, and they want to run through the list of topics. They want their managers to respond in the same way, and on time. Understanding this, the members of the leadership team are able to respond accordingly. As a result we are training the physician leaders, nursing leaders, and other staff members in the concepts in order to improve communication with our patients and enable us to work more effectively across the various business units. We believe this will improve our quality and service metrics and will have the ultimate result of benefiting us financially.

This book describes these concepts succinctly. It contains true stories that exemplify how healthcare professionals have used the concepts to improve patient safety by helping staff members get their motivational needs met daily. In this way they keep themselves out of distress, significantly reducing the number of preventable medical errors. The book also describes how healthcare providers can increase patient satisfaction by communicating with patients in their preferred mode and by helping patients get their motivational needs met during their hospital stay and in visits to clinics and doctors' offices.

Healthcare professionals have known for years that people can avoid the onset of many of the leading causes of premature death—for example, heart attacks, stroke, and diabetes—if they lead healthy lifestyles, exercise, and lose weight. Nearly every healthcare professional has tried unsuccessfully to persuade his or her patients to adopt a healthy lifestyle and is frustrated by the fact that people refuse to do it. Chapter 10 contains specific strategies, individualized for each of the six personality types, that healthcare providers can use to accomplish this.

This book is a welcome addition to the medical literature because it outlines the concepts of a tool that provides the ultimate safety. Listen to what people say and how they say it. Respond not only with empathy but with words and phrases that resonate with your listener.

Hugh Tappan
CEO, Wesley Medical Center
Wichita, Kansas

Acknowledgments

We are deeply indebted to all those who have contributed to this book. We especially want to thank Dr. Taibi Kahler, whose genius resulted in many of the discoveries that led to the concepts described in this book. The power of the concepts of Dr. Kahler's Process Communication Model® has enabled executives to lead their organizations more profitably; managers to operate their organizations more effectively; healthcare professionals to reduce human error, thereby improving patient safety and both patient and staff satisfaction; and educators to individualize the way they teach so that they reach and motivate every student, thereby reducing disruptive behaviors in the classroom and improving student academic achievement. In addition, Dr. Kahler's Process Therapy Model™ has enabled psychiatrists and psychologists to greatly reduce the treatment time of their patients and speed up their recovery.

For more than 40 years, Dr. Kahler's discoveries have enriched the lives of people in all walks of life. We have enjoyed our association with him for more than 25 years. He has changed our lives, and his Process Communication Model® has enabled us to be more effective leaders in every organization we have headed. More important, the concepts of Process Communication have enabled us to improve the lives of all those with whom we interact every day and have enabled us to positively impact professionals, leaders, teachers, students, and educators throughout the country.

We also are indebted to the many people who shared stories with us detailing the ways they have used the concepts. We especially want to thank the doctors, nurses, and other health-care professionals who described how they use the concepts to treat patients, to reduce conflict and promote teamwork within their facilities, and to improve patient safety and patient and staff satisfaction. We also want to thank the patients who shared their stories—both positive and negative—with us. Some of those who provided stories are named in the book. Others are not, at their request. All the stories are true.

We especially are grateful to Andrea and Werner Naef, directors of Kahler Communications Oceania, and Dr. Brad Spencer, CEO of Spencer, Schenk, Capers, for introducing us to some of their clients and persuading them to provide stories for the book. We also want to thank Nate Regier, PhD, founding member partner of Next Element Consulting, for introducing us to Dr. Hugh Tappan, who wrote one of the forewords in this book. We greatly appreciate and are indebted to Dr. Janet Hranicky, founder and president of the American Health Institute, for sharing with us the results of her more than 30 years of research with cancer patients.

We want to thank all the doctors, nurses, and physical and occupational therapists who have taken such excellent care of us throughout our lives. They have provided outstanding care and medical advice and have kept us alive and ambulatory so that we could continue to train professionals and others in the concepts contained in this book. They literally saved the life of one of the authors, Joe, when his femoral artery ruptured.

Finally, we want to thank Matt Meinholz of the ASQ Quality Press for his foresight in recognizing the value of this book and for encouraging us to write it. We also want to thank the other ASQ staff members who worked with us. We especially are indebted to the staff of Kinetic Publishing Services, LLC, for editing and typesetting the book. This is a better book because of their expertise, suggestions, and corrections.

To all of them we say a sincere and heartfelt thank you. This book would not have been possible without their help.

Introduction

*E*stablishing a Culture of Patient Safety: Improving Communication, Building Relationships, and Using Quality Tools aims to provide a road map to help healthcare professionals establish a culture of patient safety in their facilities and practices, provide high-quality healthcare, and increase patient and staff satisfaction by improving communication among staff members and between medical staff and patients, by describing what each of six types of people will do in distress, by providing strategies that will allow healthcare professionals to deal more effectively with staff members and patients in distress, and by showing healthcare professionals how to keep themselves out of distress by getting their motivational needs met positively every day.

The concepts described in this book are based on science and have withstood more than 40 years of scrutiny and scientific inquiry. They originally were used as a clinical model to help patients help themselves, and, indeed, they still are used in this manner. The originator of the concepts, Dr. Taibi Kahler, is an internationally recognized clinical psychologist who was awarded the 1977 Eric Berne Memorial Scientific Award for the clinical application of a discovery he made in 1971. That discovery enabled clinicians to greatly reduce the treatment time of patients by lessening their resistance as a result of miscommunication between them and their doctors.

Dr. Terrance McGuire, the consulting psychiatrist for the NASA space program for more than 40 years, was so impressed by Dr. Kahler that he invited him to participate in the 1978 round of astronaut selection interviews. Dr. Kahler's involvement with the space program led him to turn the concepts into a behavioral model. When CEOs heard about the concepts, they asked Dr. Kahler to translate the model into management and leadership terms. He did, and in 1981 he developed a commercial model that is being used in healthcare facilities, corporations, nonprofit organizations, and other organizations around the world to help increase employee productivity, job satisfaction, morale, and corporate profitability. In healthcare facilities, these concepts have enabled healthcare professionals to greatly reduce accidents (including accidental deaths), improve patient safety and satisfaction, and improve staff satisfaction and retention. Since 1986 the model also has been used in education to help teachers individualize instruction so that they reach and teach every student more effectively.

The concepts are universal; that is, they apply in every culture. They have proved to be effective everywhere they are used—in the United States, Canada, Europe, Asia, Australia, New Zealand, Africa, Latin America, and the Caribbean. Included in the book are stories from several healthcare professionals and healthcare organizations in the United States, Canada, Europe, and New Zealand. Many healthcare professionals have told the authors that being able to apply these concepts to their patients and their colleagues has enabled them to establish positive relationships with all their patients and to deal more effectively with patients and caregivers in distress. Former president William Clinton told the authors in 1997 that he considered Dr. Kahler to be a genius. President Clinton used the concepts in his speeches, and Dr. Kahler served as a psycho-demographer during Clinton's presidency.

But improving patient safety and satisfaction is only one aspect of improving the quality of healthcare. To improve healthcare in the United States we also must take a proactive approach by encouraging people to lead healthier lifestyles, thereby reducing the likelihood that they will develop diabetes, suffer heart attacks or strokes, or develop other conditions that will require hospitalization or medical treatment. Ultimately, the responsibility of eating better, exercising, and pursuing healthy lifestyles is theirs. The question is, how can healthcare professionals persuade people to live healthier lifestyles? Chapter 10 provides specific strategies for accomplishing this.

The concepts outlined in this book will enable doctors and others to improve the teamwork in their facilities, improve the safety and satisfaction of their patients, enable facilities and partnerships to retain highly qualified staff, and persuade people to lead healthier lifestyles. In addition, if people learn how to get their needs met at home and in their place of work every day, they will be happier, healthier, and more productive. They also will be more likely to pursue a healthy lifestyle.

The concepts are explained in the first part of the book. Several examples illustrate how doctors, nurses, and administrators have used the concepts to reduce human error, improve patient safety, and improve doctor and patient satisfaction. Also included are stories illustrating how patients who understand the concepts have used them with their doctors to reduce the chance of human error. All the stories are true. The last two chapters of the book discuss ways that doctors can use the concepts to persuade their patients to lose weight and lead healthier lifestyles, and to lead their staff members to embrace the need to reduce preventable medical errors and improve the quality of patient care.

One of the authors, Joe Pauley, first learned of the concepts as a management tool when working for the US government. He used the concepts to increase productivity and employee and customer satisfaction in every department he headed. For the past 23 years he has used the concepts in leading a successful international training and consulting company and in helping people at all levels in healthcare facilities improve patient safety and satisfaction, and improve staff productivity and organization profitability. He also has helped people at all levels in corporations, government, nonprofits, and education improve the productivity and profitability of their organizations.

The other author, Judy Pauley, used the concepts in leading the science departments of a high school where she taught chemistry and physics, in leading several scientific organizations, and in inspiring her chemistry and physics students to pursue careers in various science and engineering fields. She was named Science Teacher of the Year three times. For the past 17 years, she successfully led her company in helping educators reach and teach every student.

The Pauleys are the recipients of the 2008 Individual Crystal Star Award from the National Dropout Prevention Network at Clemson University. The award acknowledges their work in helping educators apply the concepts in their classrooms to reach and teach every student in order to prepare them for work in the twenty-first century. Judy can be reached at judy@kahlercom.com. Joe can be reached at joe@kahlercom.com.

Enjoy the book.

1

The Need to Improve Patient Safety

"Have you seen this morning's paper? They replaced the wrong hip at the Washington Hospital Center yesterday. I got the right one for you. Of course, I had a zipper on the other one to show me which one I should be working on." This is how an orthopedic surgeon in Maryland greeted one of the authors the morning after he replaced the author's left hip. Was this mistake at the Washington Hospital Center an unusual occurrence, or are mistakes in healthcare facilities fairly common?

Millions of patients receive high-quality healthcare every year. Unfortunately, preventable medical errors occur, and they occur fairly often. For example, a surgeon in a Florida hospital amputated the wrong leg of a patient. In the state of Washington, a heart transplant patient received a heart with the wrong blood type. In a Boston hospital, one doctor simultaneously was overseeing blood transfusions for two patients undergoing operations and switched the different blood types. In another instance, an anesthesiologist forgot to turn the anesthesia on after paralyzing the patient during an orthopedic operation. The patient was awake throughout the operation. She tried to signal the surgeon, but was unable to because she was paralyzed. She subsequently sued the anesthesiologist.

In another hospital, a patient went in for a routine surgical procedure. The anesthesiologist had difficulty administering the anesthetic and decided to intubate the patient. He was not able to do so at first, but continued to try even though the patient's condition deteriorated. He ignored suggestions from one nurse that the "trachy machine" was available. He also ignored the suggestion of another nurse that there was a bed available in intensive care. Finally he gave up and decided to revive the patient. They were unsuccessful and finally rushed her to intensive care. She remained in a coma and died 13 days later without ever regaining consciousness. We will discuss this example in more detail in the chapter on distress (Chapter 8).

According to a report by the Institute of Medicine (IOM) that quoted estimates from two major studies, between 44,000 and 98,000 preventable medical deaths occur in healthcare facilities in the United States each year.[1] A study published by HealthGrades in March 2011 found that from 2007 through 2009, 52,127 Medicare inpatients developed hospital-acquired bloodstream infections, and 8,114 of them did not survive their hospitalization. The study also reported that in the same period there were 708,642 total patient safety events affecting 667,828 Medicare beneficiaries and there were 79,670 patient deaths among patients who experienced one or more patient events.[2] According to a World Health Organization report, 1 in 10 individuals receiving medical care will suffer preventable harm.[3] A study by the IOM found that 1.5 million Americans are injured by a medication error every year.[4] According to the Centers for Disease Control, there are 2 million acquired infections in hospitals in the United States every year.[5] It is estimated that medical errors cost between $17 billion and $29 billion annually. Clearly, this is not acceptable and has to be improved.

In a recent article published in the *New England Journal of Medicine*, researchers report that there was no significant improvement in patient safety in the 10 years since the IOM published its report *To Err Is Human*. The researchers studied 10 hospitals in North Carolina from 2002 to 2007 and found that medical harms remain common, with little evidence of widespread improvement. They also found there was no significant improvement in patient safety from year to year. They concluded, "Further efforts are needed to translate effective safety interventions into routine practice and to monitor health care safety over time."[6]

Although the number of patients who die is a relatively small percentage of the millions of patients who are treated successfully every year, the object is to reduce the number of errors to as close to zero as possible. The question is how to reduce the number of these errors and improve patient safety and satisfaction.

By using checklists and quality tools and by collecting data on the various processes in healthcare facilities, healthcare providers can improve the processes to reduce errors. For example, at Suburban Hospital in Bethesda, Maryland, a patient had 80% blockage in two arteries. A doctor used the femoral artery to access the arteries in order to emplace the stents to keep the arteries open. After the operation, a nurse in the cath lab briefed the patient on what he needed to do to keep from rupturing the artery, including the need to avoid straining when he went to the bathroom. The patient followed her instructions faithfully and was looking forward to a complete recovery. Two days later the patient was taking a soft drink from a plastic carton when the plug loosened and the femoral artery ruptured. The patient was readmitted to the hospital. The next morning the nurse from the cath lab visited the patient to debrief him on what happened to cause the rupture. After the patient explained what had happened, the nurse said she would include that in her briefing from then on so that other patients could benefit from his experience. The patient was impressed and told the nurse so. She replied that she used the quality tool PDSA (plan, do, study, act) every day to improve patient safety at the hospital. She added that the hospital was committed to continuous improvement in developing a culture of patient safety.

At Inova Mount Vernon Hospital in Mount Vernon, Virginia, patients were spending too much time in the emergency department because of process inefficiencies. To eliminate dissatisfaction among patients and the community, the hospital used quality tools to strengthen the emergency department process and reduce patients' length of stay by nearly two hours. According to the article "On the Clock," by Robert Q. Watson, a senior associate at Healthcare Performance Partners (a lead healthcare consulting company), and Ken Leeson, the executive director of process improvement at Inova Health Systems in Falls Church, Virginia, the time that had elapsed from when a patient entered the emergency department to the time the patient was discharged was two hours longer than that at the best emergency departments in the United States.[7]

Because of the delay in service, neither the patients nor the community was satisfied with the emergency room, and many left the hospital before being seen by a doctor. The hospital decided to review its procedures and look for ways to reduce the length of stay while still providing high-quality healthcare. The hospital set a goal of reducing the patient's length of stay from 266 minutes to 125 minutes, using quality tools such as abbreviated kaizen events, value-stream mapping, metric definitions with regular reporting, brainstorming, and control charts. The hospital made great progress toward achieving its goal: Length of stay was reduced from 266 minutes to 135 minutes, patient satisfaction increased significantly, and the number of patients leaving the emergency department without being served dropped by 75%. It has not yet reached its goal of 125 minutes, but it is looking at steps it can take to reduce the time even further.

According to the article, communication within the emergency department, among departments, and among hospital administrators was very important in enabling the hospital to reduce the length of stay. Many other books explain the use of quality tools in healthcare. This book will address the communication aspects of improving quality of healthcare, patient safety, and patient satisfaction and will offer suggestions to help healthcare providers establish a culture of patient safety in their facilities. As was illustrated in the Inova example, quality tools and communication go hand in hand in accomplishing the goal of sustained high-performance healthcare.

To be effective communicators, healthcare professionals must understand the personalities of their colleagues, how they perceive the world, how they communicate, and how they are motivated. They must ensure that all staff members of the facility get their psychological needs met every day so that they are capable of thinking clearly. They also must ensure that they themselves get their motivational needs met every day so that they are able to think clearly and deal positively with the many stressful situations they encounter each day. In her excellent book *High Performance Healthcare: Using the Power of Relationships to Achieve Quality, Efficiency and Resilience*, Dr. Jody Hoffer Gittell discusses the need for "relational coordination," which she defines as "the coordination of work through relationships of shared goals, shared knowledge, and mutual respect."[8]

Dr. Gittell conducted extensive studies in the orthopedic departments of nine nonprofit hospitals in three urban areas (Boston, New York City, and Dallas) and was able to quantify the improvement in patient safety and in patient and staff satisfaction when healthcare professionals established these relationships. Specifically, she found that relational coordination resulted in a 33% reduction in length of stays in hospitals, significant increases in the quality of service, a 26% increase in postoperative freedom from pain,[9] improved surgical performance, higher patient-perceived quality of care, a savings of $670 per patient stay, a 60% reduction in patient readmissions in 7 days, a 69% reduction in patient readmissions in 30 days, improved clinical outcomes, and improved job satisfaction among care providers.[10] She documented other significant benefits as well.

Improving relationships involves more than having each member of a healthcare team talk with one another and with his or her patients. It includes individualizing the way each member of the team talks with the other members and with his or her patients. It also includes each member helping every other member and also his or her patients get their motivational needs met positively every day so that they stay out of distress and are able to think clearly and function more effectively. It also involves recognizing the symptoms of distress and providing appropriate antidotes to keep themselves and others out of distress.

This may sound like a daunting task, but it is not. However, learning this new skill will take some practice for healthcare providers to become fully proficient in applying the concepts in this book. The rewards for applying these concepts in healthcare facilities will be well worth the effort because everyone will be happier, healthier, and more productive. If healthcare professionals establish relationships with their patients, patient satisfaction will improve. If they have relationships with both their colleagues and their patients, patient safety also will improve. To establish these relationships, they must understand how their patients perceive the world, how they prefer to communicate, and how they need to be motivated. Then they must individualize the way they communicate with each patient and help their patients get their needs met when in their care. In doing so, their patients will be happier with their caregivers and with the staff of the healthcare facility.

This is especially important today because of the new procedures that healthcare providers and facilities are, or soon will be, required to follow. Dr. Ed Bujold, a family practice physician in North Carolina, told the authors that in a recent study involving Medicaid patients discharged from North Carolina hospitals, he and his colleagues found that 20% of the discharged patients had errors in their medication regimens that were serious enough to lead to hospital readmission within the next 30 days. Nationwide, the Medicare readmission rate one month after discharge from the hospital is 20%. In the near future, the Centers for Medicare and Medicaid Services will make readmissions to the hospital within 30 days of discharge a never event. This will be added to the many other never events for which Medicare does not reimburse hospitals. In Dr. Bujold's small hospital system, this would amount to $5 million in lost revenue per year.

Whether the healthcare institutions are the famous Mayo Clinic or Cleveland Clinic, a regional Carolina's Medical Center, or a small hospital struggling to put together a fledgling accountable care organization, communication among all the integrated participants will be paramount to the success of the organization. The financial viability of the organization is at stake in this new environment in which healthcare providers now participate.

To this end, Dr. Bujold is heading a pilot project in his own hospital system aimed at decreasing readmission rates within 30 days for Medicare patients. This is a collaborative effort involving emergency departments and emergency physicians, hospitalists, physicians in private practice, physicians employed by his hospital system, home health nurses, social workers, physical therapists, hospital administrative personnel, pharmacists, and patients. Clear and effective communication will be critically important to the success of the project.

Within this very complicated system, those who can identify symptoms that their patients are starting to get into distress or are in severe distress can intervene quickly and invite them out of distress. This will help ensure that patients hear the message and are also in a positive frame of mind. It is well documented that patients with a positive attitude recover from illnesses, injuries, and operations much more quickly than those who remain in distress. With better communication, patients are more likely to take their medication appropriately, manage their chronic medical diseases, and not be readmitted to hospitals. That benefits everyone.

Dr. Bujold believes that in the next several years, good communication within doctors' offices among doctors, employees, and patients will be paramount to the success of the practice, whether it is small or large. Tremendous pressures are pushing employees in medical office settings to the breaking point, and if these pressures are not managed effectively, Dr. Bujold predicts many older physicians will retire and a number of other physicians in the primary care workforce will be forced to work for large hospital entities. Private practice and the friendly neighborhood primary care physician may become a relic of the past. The federal government, insurance entities, and primary care organizations are now promoting care delivery systems based on National Committee for Quality Assurance (NCQA) certified Patient Centered Medical Homes (PCMHs). This certification process is much like the system that hospitals have participated in for years through the Joint Commission on Accreditation of Hospitals Organization (JCAHO).

The PCMH approach provides comprehensive primary care for children, youth, and adults. In the PCMH healthcare setting, partnerships are facilitated among individual patients, their personal physicians, and, when appropriate, the patient's family. The American Academy of Pediatrics (AAP), the American Academy of Family Physicians (AAFP), the American College of Physicians (ACP), and the American Osteopathic Association (AOA), representing about 333,000 physicians, have developed the following joint principles to describe the PCMH:

> *Personal physician*—Each patient has an ongoing relationship with a personal physician trained to provide first contact and continuous and comprehensive care.
>
> *Physician-directed medical practice*—The personal physician leads a team of individuals at the practice level who collectively take responsibility for the ongoing care of patients.
>
> *Whole-person orientation*—The personal physician is responsible for providing for all the patient's healthcare needs or taking responsibility for appropriately arranging

care with other qualified professionals. This includes care for all stages of life: acute care, chronic care, preventive services, and end-of-life care.

Care is coordinated and/or integrated across all elements of the complex healthcare system (e.g., subspecialty care, hospitals, home health agencies, and nursing homes) and the patient's community (e.g., family, public, and private community-based services). Care is facilitated by registries, information technology, health information exchange, and other means to ensure that patients get the indicated care when and where they need and want it and in a culturally and linguistically appropriate manner.

Quality and safety are hallmarks of the medical home:

— Practices advocate for their patients to support the attainment of optimal, patient-centered outcomes that are defined by a care-planning process driven by a compassionate, robust partnership among physicians, patients, and the patient's family.

— Evidence-based medicine and clinical decision-support tools guide decision making.

— Physicians in the practice accept accountability for continuous quality improvement through voluntary engagement in performance measurement and improvement.

— Patients actively participate in decision making, and feedback is sought to ensure patients' expectations are being met.

— Information technology is utilized appropriately to support optimal patient care, performance measurement, patient education, and enhanced communication.

— Practices go through a voluntary recognition process by an appropriate nongovernmental entity to demonstrate that they are capable of providing patient-centered services consistent with the medical home model.

—Patients and families participate in quality improvement activities at the practice level.

Enhanced access to care is available through systems such as open scheduling, expanded hours, and new options for communication among patients, their personal physician, and practice staff.

In Dr. Bujold's opinion, these are admirable attributes to strive for, and they certainly will provide improved, safer medical care. However, they will require quantum shifts in the manner in which primary care physicians and their staffs deliver care in the future. Healthcare providers are asking clinic personnel to make paradigm shifts in their routines and habits. This will be a time of great danger and great opportunity for many in the primary care field. Dr. Bujold believes that many organizations will not survive because of poor training in communication and management.

The central nervous system of these PCMHs will be an integrated, "meaningful use" electronic health record. Moving from a paper environment to a paperless environment is very difficult. Dr. Bujold has witnessed colleagues move from one hospital system to another over a dysfunctional transition from paper to a computer-based electronic health record. He also knows of many practices that are very dissatisfied with their electronic health record health system vendor. Communication issues are one of their main concerns.

The concepts in this book have enabled healthcare providers to improve communication with everyone with whom they interact, identify when patients and colleagues are in distress, and enable them to invite people out of distress, thereby improving patient safety and patient and staff satisfaction.

THREE EXAMPLES

A Small Hospital

In 2008, staff morale and patient satisfaction were low at an Alabama hospital. The facility had been downsized from a hospital to a clinic in 1999 and had no identity for nearly 10 years. As a result, staff morale was very low. To improve morale and improve communication, the administration had the entire staff trained in the concepts contained in this book. Teamwork improved; communication between members of the support staff and the healthcare providers improved; team documentation of processes improved; and there was greater cooperation among all staff members. In addition, the staff used these concepts to develop communication and marketing plans to help develop an identity with the community and with the staff.

According to the administrative officer, the staff members also collected data to determine whether there was an increase in staff productivity as a result of the training. They found that even though the number of primary care providers was reduced by 20%, outpatient workload in terms of simple relative value units (RVUs) increased 10% from 72,650 RVUs in FY 2009 to 78,000 RVUs in FY 2010. (The RVU was devised by the Centers for Medicare & Medicaid Services when it developed a standardized way of measuring provider productivity. The RVU is a three-part figure based on provider skills, facility costs, and time required for the procedure. The RVU for primary care is about $89.) Figure 1.1 shows the results of that study. This translated into 7800 RVUs per primary care provider. In FY 2011 the facility began measuring performance in enhanced RVUs. Under the new system, the number of RVUs increased further. In financial terms in FY 2011, each healthcare provider earned about $430,000—the highest per-provider earnings in the 33-facility system. Prior to being trained in the concepts described in this book, the facility ranked 31st out of

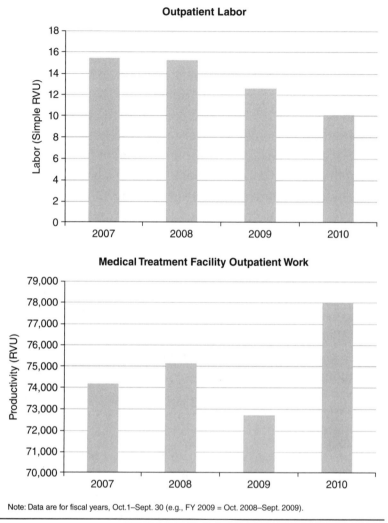

Note: Data are for fiscal years, Oct.1–Sept. 30 (e.g., FY 2009 = Oct. 2008–Sept. 2009).

Figure 1.1   Doing more with less.

the 33 facilities in the system in terms of overall performance. The facility now is the fifth-highest-ranked facility in the system in overall performance, and the staff are determined to improve further.

The hospital set an initial goal of raising patient satisfaction so that at least 85% of patients were completely satisfied with the treatment they received and with their interaction with

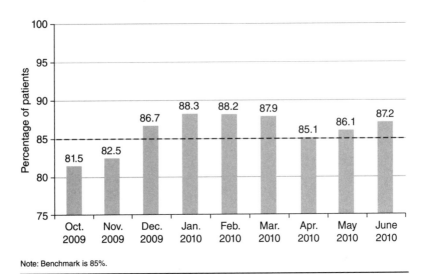

Note: Benchmark is 85%.

Figure 1.2   Courtesy and helpfulness of the staff during this visit.

members of the staff. Patient ratings of the courtesy of the staff improved each month as more members of the staff were trained. The facility met its goal of 85% patient satisfaction with the courtesy of the staff in December 2009, the month that the authors had completed training all staff members. Patient satisfaction with the courtesy of the staff continued to increase each month thereafter, reaching 88.3% in January 2010. Figure 1.2 shows the improvement each month.

During this period some staff members left the facility and were replaced by other professionals. As a result, in April 2010 patient satisfaction dipped to 85.1%. The authors trained the new staff members, and patient satisfaction rose again in the following months. In the spirit of continuous improvement, the administration raised the goal of overall patient satisfaction to 90%. According to the administrative officer, overall patient satisfaction rose to 94% in October 2010. Because of the downturn in the economy, the board of directors was planning to drastically reduce the size of the staff and the services offered. However, when the board members saw the improvement in patient satisfaction, they decided not to reduce the number of

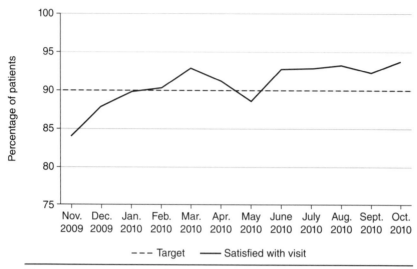

Figure 1.3   Overall satisfaction with visit.

services offered, and they reduced the size of the staff by only five positions. Figure 1.3 shows the improvement each month.

A Large Healthcare System

Ascension Health in St. Louis is the largest nonprofit healthcare facility in the United States. In 2003 it set a goal of significantly reducing workplace accidents and eliminating preventable medical deaths within five years. Using quality concepts and the concepts contained in this book, the facility greatly reduced all medical errors, including medical deaths, every year. It now recognizes that many more deaths are preventable than initially thought. This story will be discussed in more detail in Chapter 11.

A Hospital Residency Program

A doctor at a hospital in Hawaii learned the concepts of Process Communication in 2005. In 2007 he became the director of the Family Residency Program in the family medicine department of the hospital. Historically the pass rate in the department was 95%. However, the year before the doctor took over the residency program the pass rate was only 60% and the program had a sizable attrition rate. This was unacceptable to the doctor, and he decided to do something about it. He looked at the character strengths of the residents and realized all of them were quite different. They all responded to orders differently and had different strengths. Some did well checking boxes and others did not. Therefore, he decided to profile the residents and the staff members and assign as a mentor a staff member with whom the residents would relate best. He also used the profiles in assigning people to different teams.

The doctor also hired a coordinator for the program. He believed it was critically important to hire someone who genuinely cared about the residents. Therefore, he selected a person who was compassionate and warm and had great interpersonal skills. In his opinion, he had made a great choice. In working with the residents, the doctor individualized the way he communicated with them and motivated them. Some of the residents responded well to awards and praise. Others did not. Some responded better when they knew people liked them. One of the residents was very quiet and withdrawn. He preferred to be alone and tended to speak in short sentences and then only when spoken to. Also, he did not respond to any of the motivators the doctor used with the other residents. Some of the other residents were very playful, and the doctor found he had to be playful with them. He also learned that he had to set boundaries for them. He referred to the boundaries as "guard rails."

When the residents got into severe distress, the doctor told them to look at the personalized personality booklet he had given them, read the section entitled "Action Plan," and follow the strategies suggested for getting their motivational needs met positively. The pass rate increased every year until 90% of the residents were certified in 2009. In addition, no one dropped out of the program. The residents consider it to be the best residency program in the hospital, and more people apply to the program than the department can accommodate.

In his efforts to improve the certification rate of his residents, the doctor researched the personality types of those who were not getting certified. He found they were of two types— those who are compassionate, sensitive, and warm, and those who are reflective, imaginative, and calm. Interestingly, both of these personality types do not do well on tests, but for different reasons. The first type frequently experiences test anxiety. As will be explained in subsequent chapters, when they get into distress they make mistakes on things they know how to do very well. The mistakes may be silly or sometimes even tragic, and they often occur in high-stakes tests such as certification examinations. For example, in a multiple-choice test they may skip a line and mark all subsequent answers on the wrong line. As a result, all the answers after the skipped line are wrong and they fail the examination.

The second type has a difficult time with multiple-choice tests. They see so many connections between things that they think there is no one right answer. They may get into distress about it and subsequently shut down. Frequently they just sit there until time expires and do not finish the test. This type of person also may have difficulty with the oral part of the examination because he or she is quiet and tends to speak in short sentences. Again, because they see so many connections between things, they may answer the oral questions by going off on tangents and speaking in disjointed sentences. This may irritate the examiners and could lead them to believe that the resident does not understand the material.

Understanding this, the doctor made certain that all his residents got their motivational needs met the night before the examination and again in the morning before taking the exam. The different personality types, their motivational needs, their preferred mode of communication, what they will do in distress to jeopardize their work and patient safety, and proactive and reactive strategies to invite people out of distress will be explained in the chapters that follow.

2

Who Are These People?

Who are these patients, and who are the medical professionals caring for them? Dr. Taibi Kahler, a clinical psychologist and the winner of the 1977 Eric Berne Memorial Scientific Award, has identified six personality types based on how individuals take in and process information, that is, how they perceive the world. He called them Reactors, Workaholics, Persisters, Dreamers, Rebels, and Promoters. Each of the six types communicates differently, is motivated differently, learns differently, and does different things when in one of the three levels of distress.

Reactors are compassionate, sensitive, and warm. They relate to the world around them (i.e., people and things) by how they feel about them. They feel the texture of their clothes and the food they eat. They are people oriented and have great interpersonal skills. They want everyone around them to feel good, and as a result, many Reactors become nurses or doctors in order to help people recover from illnesses. They prefer to work with groups of people with whom they feel comfortable. As patients, they want to be reassured that they are good people and that the medical professionals treating them are nice people, are competent, and care about them.

Workaholics, on the other hand, are responsible, logical, and organized. They are goal-oriented linear thinkers who perceive the world through their thoughts. They thrive on data.

They think first and want others to think with them. Because they are goal oriented and think clearly, they expect others to be goal oriented and able to think clearly too. Many Workaholics become doctors or hospital administrators. As patients, they want to know that their caregivers are competent professionals who will answer their questions honestly and give them the information they want about their condition. Because they are goal oriented and willing to work hard, Workaholic patients will faithfully perform the exercises required for their recovery as long as they are reassured that their hard work is appreciated.

Persisters are conscientious, dedicated, and observant. They have high standards and a strongly developed belief and value system. They expect others to have high standards and values too. They form opinions very quickly and are quick to act on them. Because they are self-starters and goal oriented, they are driven to succeed. As a result of their commitment and determination, they frequently rise to leadership positions in an organization. One of their strengths is the ability to stick to a task they believe in until they accomplish it. Many Persisters become doctors, head hospital departments, or serve on hospital boards. As patients, they want to know that their caregivers are professional, have high standards, and are committed to quality performance. They also want to know their condition and what is required of them to recover from their illness. Once they make a commitment to do whatever is necessary to get well, they will stick to it.

Dreamers are reflective, imaginative, and calm. They see the world through reflection and think outside the box. They are very different from the other five types in that they see connections between things that the others do not see. However, before they contribute to a discussion or take action, they need time to reflect on the topic or task. When given time to reflect, they frequently are very insightful and make observations that the other types have not thought about. However, they must be given time to reflect on topics before being expected to contribute their ideas. As patients, they seldom cause problems. They want healthcare professionals to speak to them slowly, tell them to do one or two things at a time, and leave them alone to do them. They do not need a lot of personal contact.

Rebels are creative, spontaneous, and playful. They react to people and things with likes and dislikes and can have wide mood swings. They can go from love to hate in a nanosecond. They are high-energy people, are very active, and like to have fun. They are free spirits and thrive in an environment that encourages creativity and allows them freedom to express their individuality and playfulness. They are stifled by restrictions and frequently question why things have to be done a certain way. For this reason, many rebels are change agents who look for ways to make work fun and do things creatively. Some Rebels become doctors or nurses, and many become physical or occupational therapists. As patients, they want their caregivers to be lighthearted with them and treat them playfully. Rebels will do anything for people they like, and they like people who are lighthearted and fun. Therefore, to get them to do the exercises or follow the regimen necessary for their recovery, healthcare professionals should try to find ways to make the exercises fun. Some healthcare professionals speak to their Rebel patients in an upbeat and energetic tone. Others have told appropriate jokes, and some have even sung to their patients.

One of the daughters of the authors is a Rebel. She had a total knee replacement, and after the operation she went to a rehabilitation facility to regain movement in her knee. Every day she had three hours of physical and occupational therapy. She complained about the exercises the therapists had her do, especially walking around the gym with her walker. The therapists decided to make the exercises fun, so one day they had her go on a treasure hunt. They hid colored cones in several places around the gym, and she had to walk around and find them, put them in a basket, and bring them back. She walked around the gym twice picking up the cones. This was twice as much walking as she had done up to that point, and she did not complain once.

Promoters are persuasive, adaptable, and charming. They are action oriented, thrive on challenges and excitement, and make things happen. They love the challenge of selling something to someone, and they make excellent entrepreneurs because they live on the edge and respond best to short-term challenges and quick rewards. They are natural leaders because of their persuasiveness and willingness to take risk. If they go into medicine, they may become anesthetists, neurologists, or orthopedists. Some Promoters become heads of hospitals or chairs of boards of directors. As patients, they want information given to them concisely and in bullet form. They are interested in the bottom line. Tell them their condition, what they have to do to recover, what is in it for them if they follow directions, and what is the consequence if they do not.

Although everyone is one of these six types, parts of all six types can be found in everyone; however, some parts are used more often than others. Dr. Kahler describes this as a six-floor condominium with the strongest part as the base and the other parts in ascending order of dominance. Let's assume that Figure 2.1 is the profile of a male doctor. As a base Persister, he

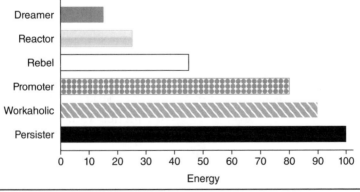

Figure 2.1 Personality components of a doctor.

is conscientious, dedicated, and observant. With Workaholic second and well developed in his personality structure, he is organized, responsible, and logical and is able to think clearly. Note that Promoter is third and also is well developed. This means that this leader is action oriented and is willing to take risks to achieve his goals.

Let's look at the impact of different personality structures from the point of view of the doctor in Figure 2.1 and a nurse who is quite different from the doctor. According to Dr. Kahler, staff members who are like the doctor in Figure 2.1 will hear his messages and understand what is expected of them. People who are not like the doctor—for example, the nurse with a personality structure like that in Figure 2.2—will not, unless the doctor communicates with the nurse in the nurse's preferred way of communicating. The doctor also needs to individualize the way he communicates with and motivates all the people with whom he interacts. This is because each of the six types is motivated differently, communicates differently, prefers a different interaction style, learns differently, and does different things when in distress; each of these will be taken up in subsequent chapters. For now, let's look at the personality structure of the nurse in Figure 2.2 and compare it with that of the doctor in Figure 2.1.

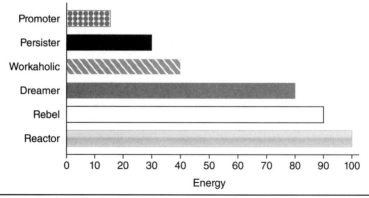

Figure 2.2 Personality components of a nurse.

This nurse is a Reactor. For the purposes of this example, we will assume the nurse is female. She is compassionate, sensitive, and warm and feels first. She has great people skills and genuinely cares how people feel; that is, she wants everyone to feel good. Completion of tasks is less important to her than working with people with whom she feels comfortable and having people like her. She has Rebel on the second floor of her condominium. Therefore, she has a lot of creativity and likes to have fun. Dreamer is her next most well developed part. As a result, she has some ability to conceptualize and see connections between things that others may not see. Workaholic is on her fourth floor and is not very well developed. This indicates that she has some ability to be logical and to think clearly, but this is not her strong suit. She is not particularly task oriented. Persister is on the fifth floor of her condominium and is the next to least well developed part of her personality structure. As a result, she does not have strongly held opinions. In fact, in elections, if she votes, she normally votes for candidates she feels are nice people and does not necessarily vote on the issues. Promoter is the least well developed part of her personality. She is not adventuresome and does not feel comfortable taking risk. She is most comfortable keeping her savings in certificates of deposit or savings accounts. If she invests in the stock market, she normally invests in ultraconservative stocks.

Most adults can energize two or three of their personality parts very easily. Most children can energize only one or two. Therein lies the problem. The doctor in Figure 2.1 energizes his Persister part most often, and he also energizes his Workaholic part very easily. He rarely ever uses the Dreamer or Reactor parts of his personality. His personality structure is almost the reverse of the nurse in Figure 2.2. As a result, the nurse may feel that the doctor does not like her, probably will get into distress about it, and, when that happens, will not hear the doctor's message or understand what is expected of her. As we will see in Chapter 8, Reactors in distress make mistakes. The mistakes can be silly or, in some instances, tragic, similar to some of the examples cited in Chapter 9.

What can the doctor do about it? The rest of this book answers that question.

Because each of the six types has different strengths, all have something to contribute to the healthcare facility in carrying out its mission. Therefore, wise administrators and doctors assess the character strengths needed to achieve the mission and deliberately seek out those persons who have those strengths.

Successful medical practitioners recognize the talents of all their staff members and know how to access those talents. However, to do this successfully, healthcare providers need to be able to communicate with and motivate each person in ways that are most effective for that individual. The following chapters will explain how to do this.

3

Interaction Styles

In his book *The Mastery of Management*, Dr. Taibi Kahler explains how each of the six types prefers to be managed and interacts with others.[11] He describes four classical management styles: the Autocratic, the Democratic, the Benevolent, and the Laissez Faire. The person using the Autocratic style gives commands and directives, and encourages others to respond directly to her or him. This is a task-oriented style and is useful with those who require direction, structure, definition, or training. The Democratic style is based on the principles of group participation and decision making. The person using this style encourages interaction between and among others, solicits feedback, and fosters independent thinking. This style also is called a participatory style and encourages goal-oriented people to grow at their own pace. This style also increases group cohesion and enhances morale by getting everyone to participate in setting common goals.

Individual feelings are more important than tasks to people who use the Benevolent style. These people assume that when people feel good, they do better work. Therefore, they foster a sense of belonging in others by interacting in a nurturing and accepting way. This style works well with people who require unconditional acceptance. However, some people dislike mixing personal and professional relationships and consider this style an invasion of privacy. The Laissez Faire style is the most nondirective of the four styles. People who use this style invite others to assume as much responsibility as they can handle. This style works well for self-styled, "do your own thing" individuals as well as people who resent authority and a lot of rules and regulations. This style invites independency and creativity; however, it does not provide the direction and structure that some people need.

To date, no single interaction style has been identified that is effective with everyone. Instead, to be effective, leaders need to use an individualistic interaction style in order to interact successfully. Workaholics and Persisters are most productive when their supervisors use a Democratic interaction or management style in which the two personality types participate in setting team goals and choosing the paths to achieve them. Reactors consider their coworkers part of their extended family and are most productive in an environment in which everyone is nurtured as if they were members of one big happy family. Rebels are most productive when their manager uses a Laissez Faire management style in which they are encouraged to use their creativity in finding innovative solutions to problems with a minimum of direction and supervision. Dreamers respond well to an Autocratic style in which they are told to do one thing at a time and are left alone to accomplish it. Promoters also respond well to an Autocratic style. Tell them the goal and the quick reward they will get for achieving it, and then get out of their way. Interacting the same way with everyone is not interacting with, or managing, them equally. Neither is it treating them fairly (see Table 3.1).

When administrators, doctors, nurses, and other healthcare professionals do not individualize the way they interact with their colleagues and patients and do not motivate each according to her or his needs, their colleagues, patients, and service providers may show predictable and observable signs of distress. Healthcare professionals who know the warning signs to look

Table 3.1 Preferred interaction style of each personality type.

Personality type	Interaction style
Reactor	Benevolent
Workaholic	Democratic
Persister	Democratic
Dreamer	Autocratic
Rebel	Laissez Faire
Promoter	Autocratic

for and who recognize the significance of the behavior when they see it can intervene quickly to remotivate the employee.

One of the neighbors of the authors had an appointment to have a spinal tap done in the emergency room of her local hospital. Many patients were being treated in the emergency room that day, and the doctors were using an Autocratic style with the nurses. Some of the nurses were not comfortable with that style and began making mistakes. The nurse who was trying to draw blood from the neighbor's arm was in such distress that she was unable to insert the needle in the patient's vein. After several unsuccessful tries, she apologized and left to try to recover her composure. The doctors continued to use an Autocratic style with the nurses, and some of them, including the nurse who was trying to draw blood from the neighbor, continued to make mistakes. The nurse tried several times to draw the blood sample but was unsuccessful. After an hour, the neighbor helped the nurse get her Recognition of Person need met by telling her that she was glad that she was the one trying to draw her blood, because she knew that the nurse cared about her patients. The nurse apologized for not being able to draw the blood successfully. The neighbor immediately told her it was OK, adding that she knew how busy everyone was and that she knew the nurse was a highly qualified professional who cared about the well-being of her patients and wanted to help them heal. The nurse immediately came out of distress. She inserted the needle into the neighbor's vein on the first try and successfully drew the blood sample. The neighbor's comment was, "My only regret is that I didn't help her get her Recognition of Person need met when she came to draw the blood the first time." How to invite people out of distress is discussed in more detail in Chapters 8 and 9. The motivational needs of the six types are discussed in Chapter 6.

In an article entitled "Why CEOs Need to Be Honest with Their Boards," Dirk Hobgood, a governance and risk-management consultant and chief financial officer at the consulting and executive search firm Accretive Solutions, was quoted as saying, "In the past, CEOs had carte blanche to do what they needed to do to run the company. Today's CEO really has to work effectively as a team member with the board and keep them up-to-date and keep the players involved."[12] In other words, the Autocratic style does not work with most boards any longer, either. Board members want to be part of the decision-making process and want the CEO to use a Democratic interaction style. According to the article, they also want CEOs to be honest with them and not try to hide or downplay problems. Indeed, when James A. Kilts, former CEO of Gillette Co. and Nabisco, addresses groups of leaders, he gives the following advice: "Tell the truth."

Only 15% of the North American population (Promoters and Dreamers) is comfortable with the Autocratic interaction style. The other 85% is not comfortable with it, and some openly rebel against it. Workaholics need an opportunity to provide information and recommend and discuss possible options. Persisters need to express their opinions and want to be heard. Rebels hate to be told what to do, and, as was illustrated in the story, Reactors often feel attacked when ordered around. Only 35% of the North American population is completely comfortable with the Democratic style (Workaholics and Persisters). Only 30% of the North American population is comfortable with the Benevolent style (Reactors), and only 20% is comfortable with the Laissez Faire style (Rebels). Therefore, if administrators want to be effective with all their staff members, doctors, and other healthcare professionals, they must use an individualistic style. The same is true for doctors and nurses. If they want to be effective with all their patients, they must individualize the way they interact with them.

In an individualistic interaction style, people match the style they use with each person to the personality type of that person. For example, with a Promoter patient, a doctor would use an Autocratic style. With a Workaholic or a Persister, he or she would use a Democratic style. With a Reactor the doctor would use a Benevolent style, and with a Rebel he or she would use a Laissez Faire style.

What would that look like? Major General (ret.) Gale S. Pollock is the former acting surgeon general of the US Army. She learned the concepts of Process Communication when she was a lieutenant colonel and was about to take over a dysfunctional department in a large army medical center. Many of the nurses in her department were Reactors, and thus they needed to feel comfortable in a nurturing environment to be effective. Therefore, General Pollock used a Benevolent interaction style with them so that they felt that they and their colleagues in the department were like members of one big happy family. General Pollock was least comfortable with this style, and it took a lot of energy for her to do this. However, it made such a big difference for the nurses that General Pollock considered it worth the energy expenditure on her part.

One of the members of her department was a Dreamer, and so General Pollock used an Autocratic interaction style with her. General Pollock directed her to do only one or two things at a time and gave her specific directives about them. She also used the Autocratic style with the Promoters who worked with her. In this way, there was no ambiguity in what they were to do and they responded well to this style. One Promoter was so impressed with General Pollock's interactions with him that he himself learned the concepts and used them in every leadership position he subsequently held.

With the Rebel staff member, General Pollock used the Laissez Faire interaction style. She told him what she wanted done and let him use his creativity to develop ways to carry out his duties. He responded well to this style and became a strong advocate for the department. General Pollock has Workaholic and Persister as the two most well developed parts of her personality, and she is most comfortable using the Democratic interaction style. Therefore, it was very easy for her to use this style with the Workaholics and Persisters on her staff and they responded well. As a result of using an individualistic interaction style, she was able to turn the dysfunctional department completely around. The army was so impressed with her success that they reached two years below the promotion zone to promote her to colonel from lieutenant colonel.

Using the individualistic interaction style required General Pollock to use a lot of energy, which was not easy at first. However, the more she used this style, the easier it became. Moreover, the results were so positive for everyone that she considers the expenditure of energy well worthwhile. Staff job satisfaction and job performance improved. Patient safety and satisfaction improved. Her superiors were delighted with the improvement, and she found great personal satisfaction in being the catalyst for the improvement. Specific examples of things she did with some of her staff members are described in other chapters.

Flexibility in communication is the key to successful interaction. People who shift personality traits to meet the personality types of others invite open and successful communication. They also establish trust. In addition, people who use a wider range of their personality guarantee themselves less emotional distress. Initially, this requires a lot of energy on the part of healthcare professionals; they must decide for themselves if the improved communication, quality, productivity, and profitability are worth the expenditure of energy. When they see the positive results, many believe it is.

According to the *Wall Street Journal* article cited earlier, CEOs who fail to change from an Autocratic interaction style to a Democratic interaction style increasingly risk being fired. In a Booz Allen study quoted in the article, nearly 32% of CEOs worldwide who stepped down in 2006 did so as a result of conflicts with their boards. The forced departures were nearly always because of transparency issues. They represent a slow deterioration of trust resulting from the inability of CEOs to communicate effectively with board members. Typically there were multiple events where the boards felt left out or felt that the CEO was leading them down the wrong path. Failure to communicate with board members also can increase company liability. In a handful of recent lawsuits, judges have sharply rebuked CEOs who made big plans without informing their boards.

Individualized and open communication is needed especially when healthcare professionals deal with the public. In "Evaluation of the Public Review Process and Risk Communication at High-Level Biocontainment Laboratories," Margaret Race discusses qualitative factors such as trust, familiarity, catastrophic potential, and individual control, which have strong effects on perceptions and levels of concern about risks. From her research she concluded, "How information is shared may be as important as what is presented about a complex project" in getting projects approved.[13] According to the researchers cited in her article, "Lack of communication and miscommunication with the public are major factors in failure, or near failure, of projects."[14] She explains that citizen opponents of high-level biocontainment laboratories in Boston and Denver stated they were upset by the tone of their meetings and interactions with experts. They felt the experts were dismissive of their questions, considered their concerns baseless, and were telling them what would be done rather than discussing public concerns. They also expressed offense at being talked down to by "arrogant, condescending experts."[15]

Dr. Constance Battle provided an example of arrogant healthcare professionals in the birth of her daughter Ursula. At 5:00 a.m. Dr. Battle went into labor. The doctor did an amniotomy, which is contraindicated for a breached baby. He then ordered an X-ray, which indicated that the baby was in a breached position. He said, "You know the baby is in the breached position." At that point the doctor tried oxytocin, which is against the rules for a first delivery in an untried pelvis. He left the bedside without determining that the oxytocin drip was at the appropriate frequency and strength. Instead, he left that determination to a nurse who had returned that day from a nine-year maternity leave. The nurse gave Dr. Battle oxytocin by mouth, which is contraindicated and against ACOG (American College of Obstetricians and Gynecologists) guidelines.

Dr. Battle began to experience frequent and massive tetanic contractions and asked for her husband and the doctors. The nurse refused to get them, saying, "This is what having a baby is all about." The doctor returned later and did an epidural (spinal anesthesia) too early in the delivery process so that the process was slowed down. This also was contrary to accepted procedures. As labor progressed, the doctor administered a second epidural and went into the delivery room. Dr. Battle saw a look of panic on the doctor's face. The baby's bottom had come out first, but the head did not come out and there was a lack of oxygen. At that point the doctor realized he had forgotten to turn off the oxytocin. As the delivery progressed, the uterus, which was wrapped around the baby's head, was cutting off the oxygen, similar to what the frequent tetanic contractions had done.

At this point, a fourth-degree tear occurred from the mother's vagina to her rectum. With the baby still not coming out, the doctor instructed the nurses to stand on either side of the mother and push on her stomach with their elbows. As a result, Dr. Battle got documented pneumonia. The baby came out but did not begin to breathe spontaneously until 20 minutes after the delivery. Within 24 hours the baby manifested seizure activity.

By the time the baby was four months old, it was clear that she had spastic tetraplegia (cerebral palsy). In subsequent conversations with the mother, the doctor called the baby a "pumpkin head." The parents sued the hospital and won. During the trial, it was established that the doctors had dismissed their own established procedural guidelines. They displayed desultory behavior during a time when not many patients were being treated in the hospital, there was arrogance during the operation and afterward, and there were eight major violations of accepted practice and considerable obfuscation.

How can healthcare professionals use the concepts of Process Communication in dealing with the public? Race provides several suggestions. According to her research, the public's overwhelming concern is trust. How can administrators gain that trust? Race says that her research shows that in those instances when the public was kept fully informed, including accurate information about accidents that occurred at the laboratory, minimal resistance occurred. The resistance was greatest in those instances where administrators withheld information, tried to maintain secrecy about the project, and treated representatives of the public arrogantly and dismissively. According to Race, "Repeatedly when information was withheld, dialogue began poorly and rarely improved without extensive work."[16]

In a hospital in Montgomery County, Maryland, the board of directors foresaw that there would be a need to expand the hospital as the population in the area grew. In the 1940s the board endorsed a long-range plan to purchase several houses adjoining the hospital property and rent them out until the time when the hospital needed to expand. In 2007, the board agreed that the time for a major expansion had arrived, and the hospital filed a proposal with the county government to expand the facility. Many of the residents in the vicinity were not happy with the plans and they objected. However, the hospital administrators were open in providing information about the need for the expansion and their plans. The county planning board held several hearings and eventually approved a modified version of the plan. The hospital did not get everything it wanted, but it got the approval to proceed with the expansion. If it had not communicated openly with everyone, it would not have been successful.

Open communication is needed in all interpersonal relationships—administrators with employees, employees with administrators, politicians with the public, family members with one another, teachers with students, and friends with friends. It is especially true for doctors and nurses dealing with patients. People do not want to be talked down to by "arrogant, condescending" people. Indeed, many patients have changed doctors not because of the doctor's competence but because they did not feel comfortable with him or her. Frequently they attribute this to the doctor having a poor bedside manner. But what they really are saying is that they are not comfortable with the interaction style the doctor uses with them.

The Autocratic style does not work with most people, including staff members in healthcare facilities. Many staff members want an opportunity to express their views and be heard. Everyone wants to be engaged in the interaction style with which they are most comfortable. When administrators and other healthcare professionals interact with people using styles that people are not comfortable with, people (and sometimes the administrators) get into distress. Chapters 8 and 9 discuss in more detail what happens when people are in distress.

4

Perceptions

As noted in Chapter 2, each of the six personality types communicates differently. This means that there are six different versions of every language. For example, if everyone speaks a common language, say English, there are six distinct versions based on the perceptions of the six types. They are so different that they may be considered separate languages. If healthcare professionals want to communicate clearly with all their patients or their colleagues, they must speak all six languages at some time. For example, several years ago the authors used to have several of the same doctors. Joe thought one of the doctors was terrific because the doctor spoke Joe's language. He did not speak Judy's language, however, and as a result, she changed doctors. The reverse situation happened with another of their doctors. Judy thought the doctor was wonderful, but Joe came home after one visit and said he was never going to see that doctor again. He subsequently switched to a different doctor. As mentioned earlier, when patients say that certain doctors have "no bedside manner," what they really are saying is that the doctor does not speak their language.

These languages are so different that it is like traveling to a foreign country, for example, Germany. If the healthcare giver wants to go to Germany and the people do not speak English, the healthcare giver must be able to speak German if he or she wants to be understood. The visitor might use an interpreter, but then he or she is dependent on the competence, understanding, and integrity of the interpreter to be certain that her or his message is conveyed accurately, interpreted correctly, and understood completely. Learning six versions of a common language may seem to be a daunting task. Fortunately, it is not. This chapter provides the framework for healthcare professionals to be able to use all six languages whenever they want. There are two aspects to this: (1) the language of perceptions and (2) the preferred channel of communication of each of the types. The first aspect is discussed here, and the second aspect will be discussed in Chapter 5.

THE LANGUAGE OF PERCEPTIONS

As noted in Chapter 2, each of the six types perceives the world differently. Reactors perceive the world through their emotions. They take in people and things through feeling for and about them. They want to share their feelings with others, and they want others to share their feelings with them. Workaholics, on the other hand, perceive the world through thoughts. They are data oriented and seek information. They want to give and receive information, and they want people to think with them. Many Workaholics and Reactors work in healthcare. Let's assume a doctor is a Workaholic and a nurse is a Reactor. The Workaholic doctor speaks the language of Thoughts and gives a lot of factual information. He wants the nurse to think with him. The Reactor nurse is most comfortable speaking the language of Emotions and wants the doctor to feel with her. This frequently results in miscommunication, with the nurse not clearly understanding what the doctor wants her to do, getting confused, and making mistakes.

Reactor patients want their healthcare professionals to spend time talking with them and listen to their feelings. Workaholic doctors who do not have the Reactor part of their personality well developed may not speak the language of Emotions and may not understand the need to do this. They want to give the patient the information they need to get well, and move on to the next patient. As a result, the patient may be dissatisfied with the doctor, regardless of the doctor's competence, experience, and professionalism.

This is also true in marriages. Workaholics and Reactors frequently marry each other. The Reactor spouse (for example, the wife) wants the Workaholic spouse to feel with her, and the Workaholic spouse wants the Reactor spouse to think with him. Friction often results because of their different perceptions of the world and because they speak different languages.

Persisters perceive the world through their opinions. When they get information, they quickly make a value judgment. They have an opinion about nearly everything, and they expect people to ask their opinion of things. Many Persisters go into the healthcare profession, and they often encounter friction in their relations with colleagues because of the different languages they speak. For example, in a hospital in Maryland, a nursing supervisor was having difficulty communicating with a Rebel nurse. The supervisor spoke the language of Opinions, and the nurse spoke the language of Reactions. As a result, they frequently misunderstood each other and began to dislike and distrust each other. Once the administrator learned the different languages, she began to communicate with the nurse in the language of Reactions. Their relationship improved immediately and they began cooperating to improve patient care and satisfaction.

Persisters tend to marry Reactors or Workaholics, and again friction results from the different perceptions of the world around them and the different languages they speak. The Persister spouse speaks the language of Opinions and expects the Workaholic or Reactor spouse to understand that language and respond to it. When that does not happen, the Persister spouse gets frustrated, frequently gets angry, and attacks the Workaholic or Reactor spouse. This is mentioned here because it may result in healthcare professionals coming to work in distress, which can have disastrous results in a healthcare facility (as we will see in Chapter 9). It also may contribute to patients arriving for medical appointments in distress. What each of the six types does in distress, and strategies for dealing with this distress, will be described in Chapters 8 and 9.

Dreamers perceive the world through inaction or reflection. They tend to reflect on subjects before speaking and usually speak slowly and deliberately when they do speak. They tend not to undertake a task until told to do so. This frequently irritates Persisters, who form opinions very quickly, act on them immediately, and expect others to do the same. It also irritates Workaholics, who frequently multitask and are very good at processing large quantities of data very quickly.

Rebels perceive the world through their reactions. They let everyone know what they like and what they do not like, usually without regard to the consequences. This frequently irritates Workaholics and Persisters, who may think that the Rebel is not taking her or his work seriously and is not committed to providing quality patient care. This is what was happening with the Persister administrator and the Rebel nurse mentioned earlier. Reactor colleagues may feel that the Rebel does not appreciate them.

Promoters perceive the world through action. They act first, usually without thinking about the consequences of their actions. They want people to act with them, and they get impatient when people engage in prolonged discussions. They want information succinctly and in bullets. They do not speak the languages of reflection or Emotions; they get impatient with a lot of unnecessary data and are not interested in the language of Opinions.

Everyone speaks the language of the perception of their base personality type fluently, and the language of the perceptions of the types on their second and third floors fairly well. Therefore, they communicate fairly well with the personality types on the bottom two or three floors of their personality condominium. They generally are much less comfortable with the languages of the personality types that are less well developed in their structure, and they probably do not understand the language of the personality types on the fifth and sixth floors of their condominium. Understanding this, it is easy to see how misunderstanding and friction arise between all these types in healthcare facilities, in marriages, and in every other walk of life. They perceive the world differently and they speak different languages.

For example, a former army nurse was a Rebel. Her immediate supervisor was a Persister with Workaholic on the second floor of his personality condominium. The Rebel spoke the language of Reactions. The Persister had Rebel on the fifth floor of his condominium and spoke only the languages of Opinions and Thoughts. Therefore, he interpreted her attempts to be lighthearted and creative as being frivolous and not dedicated to the care of her patients. He did not appreciate her candid expression of what she liked and did not like, or her attempts to do things in more creative and fun ways. Consequently, he gave her an unsatisfactory evaluation on her annual appraisal. The nurse decided she had to learn the languages of Opinions and Thoughts and stop speaking her favorite language if she was going to survive in her career. She did, and her subsequent evaluations improved. Eventually she rose to the rank of colonel before she retired.

Dr. Patch Adams told the authors he experienced a similar situation when he was in medical school. The hospital administrator, a Persister, did not speak his language and did not appreciate his humor or creativity. As a result, they frequently miscommunicated. After Dr. Adams earned his medical degree, he founded several hospitals in the United States and abroad. He uses humor and the languages of Reactions and Emotions to help heal many patients. For example, he and many of his colleagues dress as clowns when seeing patients. He has written several books in which he describes himself as a clown and describes his creative methods.

Healthcare professionals can identify the perception and personality types of people with whom they want to communicate by listening to the words they use in communicating with others. Because people also use their favorite perceptions in their writing, people in healthcare facilities can also look at their written material.

As we saw, Reactors speak the language of Emotions. A Reactor officer in one government agency used this language in writing guidance papers for subordinate offices around the country. She always told them how wonderful they were instead of focusing on the subject on which she was providing guidance. When she did provide guidance she preceded it with "I feel that . . ." Her Persister boss spoke the language of Opinions. He repeatedly told her to stop telling them how wonderful they were and concentrate on providing guidance. He usually added, "I believe you should tell them your opinion of . . ." (whatever they proposed doing). The officer usually responded by telling her boss what she felt. As their relationship deteriorated, she began to get into distress. Reactors in distress make mistakes, and many have accidents. She began to have frequent automobile accidents. After learning about the different perceptions, the boss understood why she spoke and wrote as she did, and he began speaking the language of Emotions with her. He asked her how she felt about things instead of asking her opinion of things. As a result, her morale improved, and she did not have any more accidents. Chapters 8 and 9 will discuss what the six types do when they are in distress and will provide strategies healthcare workers can use to invite them out of distress.

If healthcare professionals speak only the language of their favorite perception, they are inviting everyone into distress who is not comfortable with that language. If they want to be effective communicators, they have to individualize the way they speak to everyone.

When speaking to people individually it is easy to speak in one of these languages, but can it be done in a group? Yes—and without too much difficulty. The following is an example of how to do this.

Perception of Emotions (said softly)

"I always feel good when I see a patient who has been very sick recover fully and leave the hospital. I feel especially happy when they thank me for taking such good care of them."

Perception of Thoughts (said in a matter-of-fact tone)

"In one case the doctor used 37 stitches to close a wound. The patient was bleeding profusely and had lost four pints of blood."

Perception of Opinions (said in a matter-of-fact tone)

"I believe the doctor did an excellent job working with the patient. In my opinion we have one of the finest emergency room staffs in the state. I also believe that he is one of the finest emergency room doctors in the country."

Perception of Reactions (said energetically)

"I don't like it when people say we don't care about our patients and I hate it when they complain about having to wait when we take a critical patient ahead of them."

Perception of Action (said rapidly)

"When they bring a critical patient in, we swing into action. We diagnose the problem and immediately do whatever we have to do to stabilize the patient and give them the best possible care."

Perception of Inaction (said slowly)

"After we stabilize the patient, we transfer them to one of the wards or the operating room. Then we can relax a minute and reflect on what we just accomplished. Then we focus on the next patient."

Telling a story is one thing, but how can people use this technique in running meetings? The authors start every meeting like this: "I appreciate your being here on time. It shows that you care about one another. Thank you. We have a lot of important work to accomplish today. I sent you the items I have on my agenda so that you could think about them and be prepared to discuss them this morning. If any of you have something you want to add to the agenda, let me know and we will decide where it goes. We want to make sure we cover the most important items first. I figure it will take us about 45 minutes to cover all the items on the agenda. If we need more time, we can take it, but let's shoot for 45 minutes. Is that okay with everyone? Before we start, I'd like to share a funny story with you. Okay, let's get those creative juices flowing and generate some great action ideas. Let's get to it."

In this way everyone hears the entire opening message and pays particular attention to their part of it. The authors alternate using the various languages throughout the meeting to keep everyone tuned in and interested in what they are talking about. Does this work? Absolutely!

Rebels make up 20% of the population in North America, and Dreamers make up 10%. The majority of leaders and managers in many healthcare facilities do not speak the language of Rebels and Dreamers. This frequently leads to many Rebels and Dreamers being unhappy in their jobs and frequently results in friction between them and their managers/leaders. In one seminar the authors conducted several years ago, one of the participants, a Rebel, asked, "Why wouldn't everyone want to have Rebels working for them?" Another participant, a former president of a major US corporation, immediately replied, "Because you never come to work on time, you don't follow the dress code, you wear sandals instead of shoes, you are late for meetings, and you don't follow instructions. However, we know we need you, so we put up with you." This friction can be eliminated or greatly reduced very easily if everyone, especially leaders and managers, will speak the language of each of the types and individualize the way they motivate people. If leaders want to lead successfully, they must speak the languages of all the people they want to lead. Otherwise they will not be successful.

The same is true for doctors, nurses, and other healthcare professionals. If they want to communicate effectively with one another and with their patients, they must be able to individualize the way they communicate with one another and speak the perceptual language of the people with whom they want to communicate.

The other part of individualizing communication is to use the preferred "channel" of each individual. These channels are described, and their usage explained, in Chapter 5.

5

Channels of Communication

L eaders say that the key to establishing trust is to communicate clearly with your employees and staff members. They talk about keeping everyone informed, saying what you mean and meaning what you say, and always telling the truth. They also talk about giving honest and complete feedback to staff members. As we saw in Chapter 4, communicating effectively is much more than that. It involves speaking in the other person's favorite perception and also using their preferred channel of communication.

This chapter describes the other aspect of communicating effectively—the concept of channels of communication. There are four channels that are preferred by the six personality types (see Table 5.1). These channels can be compared to the channels of a TV set. For example, if a doctor or nurse is broadcasting on channel 9 and a patient or staff member is watching for the broadcast on channel 7, the patient or staff member will not hear the healthcare provider's message. If the doctor or nurse wants to ensure that the message is heard, he or she must broadcast on the channel the patient or staff member is watching.

Another analogy is a room with four doors. The patient or staff member has one door that is her favorite; whenever anyone knocks on that door, she hears that person and responds. The patient also has a door that is boarded up because she never uses it. Whenever anyone knocks on this door, the patient does

Table 5.1 Preferred channel of communication of each personality type.

Personality type	Channel of communication
Workaholic	Requestive
Persister	Requestive
Reactor	Nurturative
Dreamer	Directive
Rebel	Emotive
Promoter	Directive

not hear that person. Let's assume that the boarded-up door is the favorite door of the doctor. If the doctor knocks only on his favorite door, the patient will not hear the message and will not clearly understand what is expected of her. Let's also assume that the patient uses the other two doors only occasionally; for example, the patient uses one of the doors about two-thirds of the time and the other door one-third of the time. This means that the patient will not hear someone knocking on one door one-third of the time and the other door two-thirds of the time. If healthcare professionals want their patients or staff to hear their messages, they have to knock on the favorite door of each person with whom they interact.

If healthcare professionals use only their favorite channel, what impact will this have on the health of patients? According to various sources, about 20% of patients do not follow directions in taking medicines prescribed by their doctors. As we will see in subsequent chapters, this not only jeopardizes the health of these patients but also frequently leads to hospital readmissions for ailments that are unrelated to the condition for which the medicine was prescribed. Can this be attributed to a lack of communication between doctors and their patients? Often it can be. By individualizing the way they talk with their patients,

healthcare professionals may be able to eliminate this miscommunication or at least greatly reduce the percentage of
patients who do not follow directions in taking medications.

What are these channels, and which ones work best with
which personality types? Dr. Kahler has identified four channels of communication: the Directive channel, the Requestive
channel, the Nurturative channel, and the Emotive channel.
Another channel, the Interventive channel, is used only in emergencies when the other four channels do not work. Because this
channel is not the primary channel of choice for any of the six
personality types, it will not be described in further detail. As
listed in Table 5.1, the channels and the personality type that
prefers them are as follows:

1. The Directive channel lets the listener know exactly
   what is expected and is given as a clear command. For
   example, "Tell me what your symptoms are," "Hand me
   the scalpel," or "Make an appointment to come back
   and see me in 3 months." These commands are said in
   a matter-of-fact way without attacking or criticizing the
   other person. This channel works best with Promoters,
   who need to know the bottom line, and with Dreamers,
   who tend not to undertake an action until being given
   clear direction to do something. It does not work well
   with Reactors, Workaholics, and Persisters; if used with
   Rebels, it may result in the Rebel doing just the opposite
   of what he or she has been ordered to do.

2. The Requestive channel is used to ask for or give information. Persisters and Workaholics respond best to
   this channel. These personality types are self-motivated
   and usually know what is expected of them. Consequently, they prefer to be asked questions, such as,
   "What are your symptoms?" An example of this channel being used to give information is, "I want you to

come back and see me in 3 months." These requests are said matter-of-factly and not in a way that could be interpreted as being an attack or criticism. Some healthcare professionals may assume that everyone is open to this channel, but some people may be uncomfortable because they think they are being grilled when asked a lot of questions. A former staff member of one of the authors is one of them. One day when talking with the authors about the various channels, she said, "Now I know why I hate to come to your office. All you ever do is grill me." The authors immediately changed the way they communicated with her.

3. The Nurturative channel is used to communicate with Reactors, who prefer soft soothing tones and gentleness. People who do not have Reactor well developed in their personality structure are not comfortable with this channel and may reject it or misinterpret what is said. An example of this channel is, "That is a beautiful suit you are wearing." A response of "Thank you" indicates that the person is comfortable with that channel. A response similar to "Same suit I've been wearing all week" indicates that the person is not.

4. The Emotive channel is the one to use with Rebels. This is a fun channel, and the speaker's tone is upbeat, energetic, and may even ring with enthusiasm. People who prefer this channel frequently use slang in speaking to each other. For example, "Hey, bro, that is one awesome suit." Unfortunately for Rebels, many people, especially Persisters and Workaholics, who may be their doctors or bosses, are not comfortable with this channel and do not use it often, if at all. As a result, miscommunication often occurs between Rebel patients and their doctors or Rebel staff members and their bosses.

Because successful communication involves two people, there must be both an offer and a prompt, clear response that makes sense in order for communication to take place. Table 5.2 lists the four channels and gives examples of what is and what is not clear communication. When healthcare professionals offer communication in one channel and get the kind of response listed in the miscommunication column, the subconscious message to the medical professional is, "I am not comfortable with that channel. Please use another channel." The message is not, "Say it again, louder." Obviously, it is better if healthcare professionals use the correct channel every time, but if they use a channel with which the listener is not comfortable, they can listen to the response and, if necessary, offer a different channel. People almost always get a second chance if communication does not take place the first time. If healthcare professionals listen to the response they get when they initiate communication in a channel, the responder inadvertently will tell them whether communication is taking place.

Table 5.2 Examples of communication and miscommunication.

Channel	Communication	Miscommunication
Directive	Tell me where the books are. In the back office.	Do you want me to tell you where the books are?
Requestive	Where are the books? In the back office.	Do you want me to tell you where the books are?
Nurturative	You always look so stylish. Thank you.	Same suit I've worn all week.
Emotive	I dig that crazy tie. Yeh, neat huh?	There's nothing wrong with my tie.

ESTABLISHING CONTACT

To establish contact and communicate effectively with patients and staff members, healthcare professionals should combine the appropriate perception with the preferred channel of the person with whom the healthcare professional is talking (see Table 5.3). In communicating with Workaholics, doctors should use the Requestive channel and address the perception of Thoughts. In other words, they should give information or ask for data. For example, "What are your symptoms?," "Where do you hurt?," "How much is this new MRI machine going to cost?," or "You have to lose a pound a week and exercise an hour every day." Workaholics will respond immediately with the information requested or, in the case of receiving information, will hear and understand the message, even if they don't agree with it. If healthcare professionals use a different channel or perception in speaking with a Workaholic, the person with whom they are speaking may get confused and not be able to answer the question or not understand what the doctor wants them to do.

Table 5.3   Preferred channel and perception of each personality type.

Personality type	Channel	Perception
Reactor	Nurturative	Emotions (Feelings)
Workaholic	Requestive	Thoughts
Persister	Requestive	Opinions
Dreamer	Directive	Inactions (Reflections)
Rebel	Emotive	Reactions (Likes & Dislikes)
Promoter	Directive	Actions

For example, in May 2010, Joe was to have an operation early in the morning. He had to report to the hospital at 5:30 a.m. Everyone at the hospital was sleepy at that hour, and Joe decided to use the Emotive channel to try to wake everyone up and bring a smile to their faces. This worked with the patients in the waiting room, but it had no effect on the person processing Joe into the hospital—a Workaholic. Joe continued to use the Emotive channel in an effort to get him to smile but was unsuccessful. Because the hospital staff member obviously was not comfortable communicating in the Emotive channel, Joe switched to the Requestive channel and asked for information. The admitting person responded, and when Joe complimented him on how efficiently he did his work, he smiled and expedited Joe's admittance to the hospital.

Healthcare professionals can use this same technique with their patients. If they speak the patient's language and help him or her get their needs met positively, their patients will be more satisfied and will sing the praises of the facility and the doctors and nurses who care for them. If healthcare providers do this when providing medication instructions, it may be especially helpful in having patients understand the instructions. If they do not do this, it is likely that their patients will misunderstand the instructions.

This explains what people mean when they say things like, "I keep pulling these levers, but they must not be connected to anything because nothing ever happens that I want to happen" or "I must be speaking Chinese. I keep telling people what I want them to do, but they don't do it."

In communicating with Reactors, healthcare professionals should use the Nurturative channel and address the perception of Emotions. For example, "How do you feel today?," "I'm sorry that you are not feeling well today," or "I want you to feel comfortable during this examination." When people use a different channel or perception—for example, asking for information or an opinion—Reactors may get confused and not know how to respond.

With Persisters, healthcare professionals need to use the Requestive channel and ask for their opinion of things. For example, "What is your opinion of this?," "What do you believe we should do?," "What do you recommend?," or "Do you believe these exercises are helping you regain your mobility?"

With Rebels, healthcare professionals need to use the Emotive channel and the perception of Reactions (i.e., discuss their likes and dislikes). For example, "I really like the way you are doing the rehab exercises," "How do you like all the attention you are getting in here?," "The attention you get in this place is awesome," or "Is there anything you don't like about the care you are getting?" Doctors and nurses also have a favorite channel, and patients can communicate with them more effectively if they use the healthcare professionals' favorite channel and perception.

A good example of this happened to Brenda Dingwall, a team leader at the NASA Goddard Space Flight Center. Dingwall had an appointment with a neurology specialist for an examination. The doctor came in after Dingwall had been waiting in the reception area for nearly an hour. From his style of dress, his high-energy entrance, and the music that was blaring from his office, Dingwall concluded that the doctor was a Rebel. The doctor initiated conversation with her in the Emotive channel. Rather than show frustration at his lack of timeliness, Dingwall replied in the Emotive channel with a story at which he laughed. They continued to use that channel throughout the appointment. Because they were communicating so well, the doctor gave her the most complete neurological examination she had ever had. The 10-minute appointment lasted an hour, and at the end of the session, the doctor said, "I like you. You are fun."

With Promoters, healthcare workers need to use the Directive channel and the perception of Actions. For example, "Tell me what your symptoms are," "Explain how the accident occurred," or "Tell me if there is anyone who can drive you home."

Dreamers can do only one or two tasks at a time and normally don't undertake an action until they are told to do something. Therefore, medical personnel need to use the Directive channel with them and tell them to do one thing at a time. For example, "Tell me one thing you are going to do to implement this new policy" or "Tell me one thing you did this morning." Healthcare professionals also can use this channel to give medication instructions and to help Dreamer patients prioritize when they take their medicines. For example, "Take your Lipitor and your Cozaar at breakfast. Take your Actos and your metformin with your dinner." Doctors might also write these instructions out for their Dreamer patients using the Directive channel.

People often use their favorite channel and perception in communicating with others, including running staff meetings and making presentations. In staff meetings this frequently results in an undercurrent of distress so that one-hour meetings last two hours and nothing gets accomplished. In these circumstances, people frequently leave meetings feeling frustrated and may complain that they hate going to meetings. This was the case at a healthcare facility in Alabama. The people running the meetings continually used their favorite channel and perception, and in the process they antagonized many of the attendees. Meetings disintegrated into sessions in which participants complained about policies, attacked one another and the administration, considered the meetings a waste of time, and complained about having to attend them. After the administrators began using all the channels and perceptions during the meetings, the participants treated one another with more respect. They also stopped complaining during meetings, which resulted in much more productive meetings.

Wes Johnston is the chief operating officer of the American subsidiary of a South African company. After attending a strategy session with the senior officers of a satellite office, he e-mailed them using the Requestive channel and thanked them for including him in the strategy session. In the e-mail, he included sentences to help the Persisters, Workaholics, and Promoters get their psychological needs met. (These needs will be explained in Chapter 6.) One of the participants sent the following reply using the Nurturative channel and the language of Emotions: "Thank you for being so open and caring." Realizing he had miscommunicated with that participant, Johnston made certain he used the Nurturative channel and the perception of Emotions with that person in all future correspondence and in personal meetings.

If healthcare administrators want to inspire their staff members so that the staff members will want to follow them and help them accomplish their vision for their facility, the administrators have to individualize the way they communicate with staff members by using the preferred channel and perception of each person. These channels also are used in the various interaction or management styles discussed in Chapter 3.

6

Motivational Needs

As we have seen in previous chapters, each of the six personality types communicates differently, learns differently, and prefers a different management style. They also are motivated differently and do different things when in distress when their motivational needs are not met. If people are not motivated according to their individual needs, they will show predictable distress behaviors that can have a disastrous impact on patient safety and patient and staff satisfaction. At the same time, these behaviors are a good warning signal to healthcare professionals that there is miscommunication between them and their patients or between them and fellow caregivers. These warning signs provide opportunities for the caregivers to change the way they interact with those people to ensure that the patients or the staff members get their motivational needs met positively. They also enable caregivers to take corrective action to stave off possible serious mistakes in treating their patients. If healthcare professionals don't understand the significance of the behavior and take no corrective action, there can be serious consequences for the patients, the caregivers, and the healthcare facility.

MOTIVATING THE SIX PERSONALITY TYPES

Workaholics

Workaholics need to be recognized for their hard work, their good ideas, and their accomplishments. They need to hear "Good job," "Well done," or "Great idea." Time is also important to them. They need to know when things are due, and they expect meetings to start and end on time. They structure their day and may get frustrated if their planned schedule gets interrupted without warning or if staff members are late for meetings. Workaholic patients appreciate being told what their schedule is for the day, that is, when they will have therapy sessions, when shots will be administered, when they can have visitors, when meals will be served, when their doctors will visit them, and so forth. They also want as much information as possible about their condition, recovery period, and so forth. They will work harder in their rehabilitation if their efforts and their progress in recovery are praised.

An Example

One of the authors, Joe, has had three total hip replacement and one total knee replacement operations. As he was being wheeled into the rehabilitation room for his physical therapy sessions, he noticed that the other patients frequently were discouraged at the little progress they were making and were ready to give up on the exercises. Joe made a point of telling each of them how well they were doing and complimented them on their progress. He frequently added that they were doing much better than he was. The patients immediately recovered their energy and increased their efforts to do the exercises. Hospital staff can get the same results if they praise the efforts of their Workaholic and Persister patients.

Persisters

Persisters need to be recognized for their accomplishments and good ideas as well, but they also need to be recognized for their commitment, dedication, and values. They would rather be respected than liked. They respond well to "Great idea," "I admire your commitment to your patients and your ideals," and "I respect the way you not only talk the talk but also walk the walk." They cannot work for an organization that does not practice what it preaches or for people they do not respect. Persister patients will not remain the patients of healthcare professionals they do not respect. They need to know that their caregivers are competent. Caregivers must show respect for their Persister patients' integrity, honesty, and values, and they must treat their Persister patients in a professional manner. To demonstrate this respect, caregivers can praise their Persister patients for their commitment to their rehabilitation and the progress they are making and can ask their opinion of their progress.

Reactors

Reactors need to know that people like them—not for anything they have done but because they are nice people. Every day they need to hear from their significant other that they are loved. In the workplace they respond well to, "I'm glad you are here. You really care about our employees/clients/patients." Administrators can help their Reactor employees get their Recognition of Person need met by spending time talking to them about whatever the Reactor employees want to discuss. Frequently this will be about family or people who are important to them. In a healthcare facility it could be about the patients. Fifteen seconds a day is the minimum for getting this need met for the Reactor, but more is better. If Reactors have not gotten their Recognition of Person need met for a prolonged period of time, they may need much more time than that.

Reactor patients need to be told that they are nice people. For example, a caregiver might say something like, "I'm glad you are my patient because you are so nice." Caregivers might also say, "I just want to thank you for being so considerate,"

"How do you feel today?," or "I'm sorry you don't feel well. What can I do to help you feel better?"

When Reactors get their Recognition of Person need met positively, they frequently will compliment the person helping them. One of the authors, Joe, was diagnosed with 80% blockage in two of his arteries. The doctors went in through the femoral artery to insert two stents to open up the arteries. The operation was successful, and the next morning Joe was released from the hospital. However, 48 hours later the plug in the femoral artery came loose and the artery ruptured. Joe went to the emergency room, and while he was being treated, he kept giving Recognition of Person battery charges to the Reactor nurse who was assisting the doctor in treating him. After a few minutes the nurse said, "You are so nice." The few sentences were enough to keep the nurse out of distress so that she was able to think clearly and work diligently to help the doctor save Joe's life.

Reactors also need sensory stimulation. They need to work and live in a cozy nestlike environment. They like flowers and plants, soft soothing music, and comfortable chairs. Reactor patients will respond very positively to healthcare professionals who help them feel comfortable and help make the environment inviting and warm. When Reactor patients get their Recognition of Person and Sensory needs met positively, they will feel better and are likely to recover more quickly from their illness or injuries.

Dreamers

Dreamers' primary motivation is to have their own private time and their own private space. In a word, Dreamers need solitude. Unfortunately, they frequently get assigned to high-traffic areas in the workplace. Healthcare professionals will be more successful in treating Dreamer patients if they speak slowly, give them a brief explanation of their condition, tell them to do one or two things, and leave them alone to do them. Because Dreamers normally do not initiate conversations, seldom cause problems, and do not carry on lengthy conversations, they easily are overlooked. Caregivers will be more successful in treating them if they remember to carry on most of the conversation.

Rebels

Rebels are motivated by having fun and by being able to use their creative energy in positive ways. They easily are bored and need at least two hours a week of playful interaction with their peers. They are the most creative employees in a hospital but frequently march to a different drummer. As we saw in Chapter 4, their need to be creative and have fun is misunderstood frequently by their Persister and Workaholic colleagues. Healthcare professionals will be more successful with Rebel patients if they are lighthearted and joke with them.

Promoters

Promoters need action and excitement, that is, a "rush." No working 30 years for a gold watch for them. They respond to challenges, and they work for short-term goals with quick rewards. They need to see how they will benefit personally from whatever they are asked to do. If they don't get their Incident need met in the workplace, they may become a disruptive member of the team and may not carry their weight in team projects. In fact, they may abandon their teammates and leave them to fend for themselves.

Ryan Kopper is an adventure recreation facilitator at Prairie View Institution, a mental health treatment facility in Kansas that serves clients in both inpatient and outpatient settings. Every Thursday he teaches self-efficacy to a group of clients. During the first few weeks, he noticed one client who did not respond in the group. He rarely spoke in the group, rarely gave his perspective, and did not seem motivated to participate in the experiential activities. He often distanced himself from the group, as if to say, "There's nothing in this for me. This is your problem to deal with."

Kopper decided the client was a Promoter who was not getting his Incident needs met positively. Therefore, he planned some activities that the clients could do independently but with enough change and action to keep a Promoter interested. The Promoter client was the first to do his project, and he smiled all the time he was doing it. He described his project to the group and, without knowing the needs of a Promoter, described himself as functioning better when he had a sense of incidence, style, and charm. Kopper was surprised because the client had never participated in this way before and also because he was describing Promoter motivators and psychological needs.

In the next activity, Kopper directed the Promoter to record on a white board the group's comments about the previous activity. The client made a significant contribution to the discussion and recorded everyone else's comments on the board. His behavior completely changed because he was able to get his Promoter needs met positively. He participated more in that one hour than he had in the previous two months. He looked more content and seemed happy to be part of the group. However, Kopper was getting more and more tired energizing the Promoter part of his personality.

Kopper is a Persister whose current motivation is that of a Rebel. Because Promoter is on the fifth floor of his personality structure, it was not easy for him to energize his Promoter part, and it took a lot of energy for him to continue to use that part for any length of time. At the end of the first hour, they took a 10-minute break. Kopper went into the office and listened to some music to get his Rebel needs met. After the break, he ran the rest of the program using the Rebel part of his personality. The Promoter client went back into his shell and did not participate. This resulted in Kopper viewing the old behavior of the patient in an entirely different light. In the past he would have had a negative opinion of the Promoter. Now he recognized the behavior as reflecting a Promoter who was not getting his needs met for a variety of reasons. With this insight, it was easy for Kopper to feel empathetic rather than irritated.

When one of the authors, Judy, was having an operation, the anesthesiologist, a Promoter, came into the pre-op room and told her, "You have nothing to worry about. I am an expert." He clearly had not gotten his Incident need met for some time, so Judy said to him, "I'm glad to know that you are the person administering the anesthesia. I feel better knowing that the person doing that really knows what they are doing." The anesthesiologist swelled with pride and walked more erect as he left the room. The operation went very smoothly.

Whenever Joe has an operation, he makes certain that everyone on the operating team gets a battery charge for her or his motivational needs before the operation. He knows the surgeon is a Persister, but he usually does not know the other members of the team. Therefore, he gives battery charges for all the needs. For example, he sings as he is wheeled to the operating room and greets everyone along the way in an upbeat, energetic way (Playful Contact). He tells everyone he is glad they are on his operating team because they have had many years of experience (Recognition of Work), they care about their patients as people (Recognition of Person), and they are committed to providing quality healthcare (Conviction). He adds that the bottom line is that he knows everything is going to be successful because they know what they are doing and thanks them in advance (Incidence). In these few sentences he has helped those who may be Rebels, Workaholics, Persisters, Reactors, and Promoters get a battery charge so that they can think clearly during the operation. So far, every operation has been successful and incident-free.

This may seem unnecessary and like overkill to many people. Perhaps it is, but why take a chance? Dr. Lawrence Levinson, an eye doctor in Maryland, told the authors that a few years ago an anesthesiologist was going to have an operation. The surgeon was very skilled; the anesthesiologist knew him very well and had participated in many operations with him. In addition, his twin brother was going to be the anesthesiologist during the operation. Before the operation, the patient wrote, "This side" in ink on his right side, drew a line where the incision should be made, and wrote "Cut here" with an arrow pointing to the line. On his left side he wrote "Not this side," and at the other possible incision site he wrote "Not here." Even though he knew everyone very well, he was not taking any chances.

Earlier, in the Reactor section, we saw how Joe helped the emergency room nurse get her motivational need for Recognition of Person met when his femoral artery ruptured. He also helped the emergency room doctor get his Recognition of Work and Incident needs met at the same time. The doctor is highly skilled and is known for his ability to deal with crisis situations. Nonetheless, he was anxious because he was worried that Joe might die. Joe had lost a lot of blood (five pints), his blood pressure was very low (less than 32), and the doctor wanted to infuse the blood into a vein in Joe's neck so that it would quickly reach his heart. However, he was having difficulty breaking the skin to insert the needle. Finally, the doctor said, "Your skin is tough. I can't break it to get the needle in." Joe already had given the doctor battery charges for his skills and his commitment to saving patients, so this time Joe replied, "I'm tough all over. I played a complete football game with a broken leg and I caught an entire baseball game in college with a broken shoulder." The doctor remarked about Joe playing baseball in college, and Joe told him he also played soccer in college. The doctor had played soccer in college, and he and Joe talked for a minute or so about the sport. The doctor relaxed and inserted the needle into the vein in Joe's neck without any difficulty.

Healthcare professionals also can help their colleagues and patients get their needs met every day. In fact, the greatest gift caregivers can give is to help one another get their needs met. If they do this, the staff members will be happier, healthier, and more satisfied with their role in the healthcare facility. They also will stay out of distress and will be able to think more clearly in performing their duties, dealing with crisis situations, and caring for their patients. This will greatly reduce medical errors and improve patient safety. If caregivers also help their patients get their motivational needs met positively, patient satisfaction will soar.

Table 6.1 shows the motivational needs for each of the six personality types. Research shows that employees of all six types can do well in the workplace when they are motivated according to their needs.[17] A working knowledge of the concepts of Process Communication enables healthcare providers

Table 6.1 Motivational needs of each personality type.

Personality type	Motivational needs
Reactor	Recognition of Person, Sensory
Workaholic	Recognition for Work, Time Structure
Persister	Recognition for Work, Conviction
Dreamer	Solitude, Clear Directions
Rebel	Playful Contact
Promoter	Incidence, Action

to understand how to motivate each of their staff or team members and their patients so that they can address the motivational needs of each type every day. To do so, healthcare professionals can ask themselves the following questions:

1. How can I provide personal recognition for the Reactor?

2. How can I give recognition for work and provide time structure for the Workaholic?

3. How can I ensure that the task is meaningful for the Persister?

4. How can I provide reflection time, space, and structure for the Dreamer?

5. How can I help the Rebels get their Playful Contact need met?

6. How can I incorporate action and excitement for the Promoter?

If healthcare providers and administrators do this, employee motivation and job performance will improve and employees will stop their negative behaviors. This will allow administrators to spend more time focusing on goals and less time putting out fires. Tom V. Savage wrote, "Learners who get their needs met in school seldom cause trouble, because doing something that interferes with getting a need met is not in their self interest."[18] Although Savage was talking about students in the classroom, his comments are equally applicable in the workplace and especially in healthcare facilities. In a discussion with the authors in August 1990, Dr. Jonathan Knaupp, a professor at Arizona State University, said, "We can give employees what they deserve or what they need. If we give them what they need, they will deserve more." This is the key to establishing relationships and to the success of every employee—helping them get their motivational needs met every day. It is also the key to helping patients maintain a positive attitude about their condition and their willingness to stick to the regimen necessary for their successful recovery. In addition, it is critically important in persuading people to embrace a quality program and to commit to working to improve patient safety and satisfaction in healthcare facilities.

In their book *First, Break All the Rules*, Marcus Buckingham and Curt Coffman describe the results of extensive interviewing done by the Gallup organization to determine the effectiveness of a workplace.[19] It found that if employees answered 12 questions positively, they worked for an effective manager in an effective organization. All the questions can be related to the needs or character strengths of the six personality types. For example, "At work do my opinions seem to count?" clearly refers to the Conviction need of the Persister. "In the last seven days have I received recognition or praise for doing good work?" refers to the Recognition of Work need of the Workaholic and the Persister. "Does my supervisor or someone at work seem to care about me as a person?" refers to the Recognition of Person need of the Reactor.

Some of the other questions refer to the strengths of each of the six types. For example, "At work do I have an opportunity to do what I do best every day?" will mean different things for each of the six types. For the Rebel it might mean the opportunity to be creative and have fun. For the Promoter it might mean a shot at leading, selling, or being involved in challenging or exciting projects. For the Reactor it might mean a chance to use his or her excellent interpersonal skills or show concern for other people. For the Dreamer it might mean an occasion to be reflective, to conceptualize ideas, and to work alone. For the Workaholic it might mean the opportunity to analyze data or work with numbers. And for the Persister it might mean the chance to work on a project that is important, will make an impact, or is challenging. Helping employees get their needs met positively greatly improves their job satisfaction, their desire to produce quality work, and their willingness to adjust to new ideas.

Major General (ret.) Gale Pollock, the former acting surgeon general of the US Army Medical Department, learned of the concepts of Process Communication when she was a lieutenant colonel and just before she was about to take over a dysfunctional department in an army hospital. Many of the nurses in the department were Reactors who were not getting their needs met. General Pollock made sure that every member of her department got his or her needs met every day and successfully turned the department around.

She continued to use the concepts throughout her career and was promoted to major general and named chief of the Army Nurse Corps. Subsequently she was named the deputy surgeon general of the army. When the army surgeon general suddenly resigned, she became the acting surgeon general of the army.

Because of a series of negative media reports about medical care in the army and drastic budget cuts to military medical stations, morale in the Army Medical Department was extremely low. To counter this, every month General Pollock sent a five-minute video to all the staff clarifying priorities and recounting all the good things that were happening. She reinforced what a good job they were doing; how valuable they were to the military; and how much she appreciated their commitment to, and performance of, their duties. She also told them that she appreciated their concern for the wounded troops and the family members left behind. Because staff members were getting their needs met, her messages were eagerly anticipated. Moreover, the messages had the desired effect on the staff. Morale soared, and staff members rededicated themselves to serving the troops and carrying out General Pollock's vision.

As we will see in Chapter 9, ensuring that people are informed and that they get their needs met every day is the key to reducing medical accidents, improving patient safety, and improving patient and staff satisfaction.

PERSONALITY PHASE

Everyone has all eight of these motivational needs, and the more of their needs each person gets met every day, the more effective they will be. However, in each person some needs are more important than others—a result of a phenomenon Dr. Kahler calls "phase." Research shows that as people go through life, many experience what Dr. Kahler calls a "phase change." Two-thirds of people in North America experience at least one phase change in their lifetime. The percentages of people who experience a phase change may be different in other cultures.[20] When people experience a phase change, they move to the next floor of their personality structure and essentially operate with a new driving force. While experiencing a phase change (phasing), people very often exhibit intense negative behaviors associated with their current personality type. After completing a phase change, a person will have new motivational needs and a new sequence of negative behaviors. This new phase can last anywhere from two years to a lifetime. To illustrate, the most important current motivation of the doctor in Figure 2.1 is that of a Promoter. The doctor still uses the Persister part of his personality structure and still prefers to communicate in the Requestive channel and speak the language of Opinions. However, he now needs excitement and action. He may sometimes act precipitously, and if he gets into distress will show a different distress sequence. These distress sequences will be explained in detail in Chapter 8.

Phasing also may be a contributing factor in many situations in life—divorce, burnout, or a midlife crisis, to name a few. When people experience a phase change, they retain and strengthen the positive attributes and behaviors associated with past phases, and many aspects of their personality remain the same. For example, the character strengths of their base personality remain the strongest throughout their lives, and their favorite way of interacting with others remains that of their base personality. Also, their favorite way of communicating and the most well developed parts of their personality remain the same, as do their preferred learning style, their perception of the world, and their favorite working style (e.g., in groups, alone, or with one other person). The concept of phasing explains how individuals can be the same person throughout their lives even though their dreams, aspirations, careers, and personal goals may change. When people experience a phase change, they experience changes in motivation and in the way they handle distress.

What triggers a phase change? According to Dr. Kahler, 99% of phase changes are the result of prolonged severe distress. The following story illustrates the impact of phase on one person's life:

> I was born a Persister. As a Persister I learned very quickly that life was serious and I took everything seriously. I developed a sense of direction, mission and conviction and was motivated by working hard and dedicating myself to causes I believed in. Values, beliefs, dedication, commitment, respect, and community service were important to me. I was active in my church and on various committees in school. This dedication to causes has been a continuous theme throughout my life.
>
> World War II broke out when I was young and I saw newsreels of bombings and napalm attacks every time I went to the movies. We frequently had practice air raid alerts in which we turned off all the lights in the house and went into the basement to be safe. My father was a neighborhood air raid warden and walked the neighborhood with a flashlight to make certain everyone was off the streets and that no lights were on in any of the houses. This made a deep impression on me. One evening the sky

was a brilliant red at sunset and my mother commented that it looked as if the sky was on fire. I concluded that we all were going to die in a fire like the soldiers I saw in the movies.

At about this time my grandfather died and my parents traveled to the funeral. I stayed with a distant cousin for several weeks and while I lived with their family, the cousin told me my parents were never coming back. I went into severe distress and began to attack people orally for their lack of commitment and dedication. Finally I dealt with my fear and moved to the next floor in my personality condominium, i.e., the Workaholic part of my personality structure. I had completed my phase change. I was still a Persister, but now I was operating in a Workaholic mode.

In a Workaholic phase, I began to be more responsible, logical and organized. I was still conscientious and dedicated and continued to work hard for something I believed in and I was still motivated by being recognized for my work. However, now time began to be important to me. Suddenly, I needed to be on time for everything. Being late was unthinkable to me. I continued to excel in school and I also began to excel in mathematics and in logical problem solving. I began college intending to major in chemistry or physics. Eventually I majored in chemistry and went on to get my PhD in physical chemistry.

After several years in a Workaholic phase, I began to get depressed because although I was getting good grades, I had no close friends. I was working very hard in my studies and was doing cancer research and also research in electro-chemistry for the US navy. I was very successful and developed the batteries used in a submarine launched rocket named SUBROC. However,

I had no close friends and I became critical of others and began to attack them for not thinking clearly and not caring about their work. Finally, I dealt with my grief and I moved to the next floor in my condominium—my Reactor floor.

In a Reactor phase I began to establish close friendships with people, including the man I eventually married. I felt very fortunate to have three children and I developed the Reactor part of my personality even more in dealing with them. My third child had special needs and I developed my compassion, sensitivity, and warmth even more in dealing with her. However, I am still a Persister and I drew on my Persister strengths in advocating for her in school and in society.

As a Persister in a Reactor phase, I wanted to help other people too; therefore, I began to teach chemistry and physics in high school and in college so that I could help students lead more successful lives. I became active in several education and scientific organizations in order to help my students and I held leadership positions in most of them. I also became active in various community organizations, especially those that helped people with special needs. Eventually I helped co-found an organization to provide a social life for people with special needs and a respite program to assist their caregivers.

Today I am the CEO of a very successful national training and development company. We do management communication training for corporations and for various government agencies, but we also show educators how to individualize instruction so that they reach every student. This is very satisfying to me. Our company helps people in all walks of life and I feel very comfortable making decisions to continue helping them succeed.

Although I was very successful in every position I ever held in my career, there were some students and others with whom I was not successful. I never understood why I was missing them. Thanks to Dr. Kahler I now understand how I missed them. More importantly I understand what I could have done to reach them. I now use these concepts very successfully to reach all of my employees and everyone with whom I interact.

AN ANESTHETIST'S EXAMPLE

A consultant anesthetist at a tertiary referral hospital in New Zealand is a Rebel in a Dreamer phase. She was working very long hours and usually was exhausted at the end of the day. Frequently she was unhappy and found herself in distress. Once she learned that she needed time to herself during the day, every day, in order to get her Dreamer phase need met, she made sure she got this time. Suddenly she was no longer so tired, and she was much happier and more effective in her work.

She also made sure she got her needs met in her private life. She told her friends and family members that she needed some time alone every day and explained that when she withdrew from them to be alone, it was not because she did not enjoy their company, but because she had reached a saturation point and had to have some alone time. Everyone understood, and her relationships with her family members and friends improved. Because she is a base Rebel, she also needed to get her need for Playful Contact met. Therefore, she made sure she did some fun things every day. She told her Persister/Workaholic boss what her needs were and stated she periodically had to have some alone time and some time to do fun things every day at work. He understood and allowed her to take the time she needed. As a result, she was much calmer at work and much more effective.

Once she found out how to get her own needs met, the anesthetist was able to help the other members of her team get their needs met. There were eight anesthetists and several trainees in her department. Many were Reactors; therefore, she talked to them in the Nurturative channel and used the language of Emotions. They were happier and more effective. When they made a mistake, she gave them a battery charge for their Recognition of Person need. They immediately came out of distress, thus avoiding compounding the problem by making more mistakes.

The anesthetist also individualized the way she communicated with patients and with their family members. She listened to how they said what they said and then used the appropriate channel and perception to communicate with them. She also helped them get their psychological needs met. The patients and family members heard what she was saying, felt she understood them, and knew that she cared about them and their recovery. This led them to realize how important their cooperation was in their recovery and the importance of their role in that recovery. They consequently felt better and cooperated more. An example of how the anesthetist used the concepts to deal with a patient's family member who was in severe distress is included in Chapter 8.

A PATIENT'S EXAMPLE

Wendy Potter is one of four partners in the Child and Welfare Clinic in Melbourne, Florida. She is a Reactor in a Workaholic phase. When she goes to see a doctor she wants information. One day, she was going to get a penicillin shot and she asked the Reactor nurse for information. Potter was concerned because when she was eight years old she had a reaction to penicillin that included more than six months of intermittent hives. In addition, at age 12 she was given a shot of penicillin by mistake when she was hospitalized for pneumonia. She had no reaction at that time, but her parents and the nurse who gave the shot were very worried.

Because of her earlier reaction to penicillin, Potter kept trying to get information from the nurse in the primary care physician's office. The nurse called her "hon" and "sweetie" but did not give her the information she was requesting. Because of the miscommunication, Potter was not happy with the nurse and considered changing physicians due to the nurse's lack of responsiveness. Her satisfaction with the doctor remained high because he freely shared information and he gave the information in her favorite channel (Nurturative). He also spent time answering her questions and getting information from her, thereby helping her get her Recognition of Person need met. She remained under his care, and a new nurse seems to have taken over her case. The new nurse is very willing to seek out any information Potter requests. As a result, her satisfaction with the doctor is very high and she remains a patient of that doctor today.

Individualizing the way healthcare professionals communicate with and motivate one another and their patients is critically important to improving patient safety and patient and staff satisfaction. Helping cancer patients get their needs met positively can play a very important role in their recovery. This is discussed in the next chapter.

7

Using the Concepts in Treating Patients

Healthcare professionals have long known that the attitude and emotional state of patients play an important role in their general health and in how quickly they recover from illnesses or operations. According to Dr. Patrick Caulfield, the authors' orthopedist, patients who have a positive outlook on life and see the glass as half full recover much more quickly and tend to be healthier than those who have a pessimistic view of life. Those who live in a constant state of distress, who feel hopeless and are in despair, frequently have complications and tend to be less healthy and lead less healthy lifestyles than those who are full of energy and excited by what is happening in their lives.

A sign in the Joint Replacement Center at Suburban Hospital in Bethesda, Maryland, reads, "A positive attitude will shorten your recovery time." To illustrate this, Dr. Caulfield told the authors that one of his former patients was an internationally famous soccer player who wanted both knees replaced simultaneously. Dr. Caulfield normally is reluctant to replace both knees of a patient at the same time, but because of the positive attitude and insistence of the soccer player, he agreed. Two weeks after the operation, the soccer player walked into Dr. Caulfield's office without a cane. His positive attitude and determination resulted in an amazingly fast recovery.

In a recent discussion with the authors, Dr. Janet Hranicky, the founder and president of the American Health Institute, said this is especially true with cancer patients. Dr. Hranicky has been treating and doing research with cancer patients for more than 30 years. She has found that in treating her patients, she must improve their mental state as well as treat their physical symptoms in order to cure their cancer. She also discovered that many cancer patients have an attitude of denied hopelessness and that it is necessary to change that attitude if she is going to enhance their health and diminish the likelihood of a recurrence of the cancer.

According to Dr. Hranicky, cancer is a disease whose medical results are accompanied by, and sometimes dominated by, an emotional reaction to the disease. Indeed, the diagnosis of cancer still evokes in many patients a sense of uncontrollability and inevitable death. According to Dr. Hranicky, the onset of the disease often bears no apparent relation to controllable factors, and the course of the disease can be unpredictable. As a result, prolonged depression is a very frequent consequence of a cancer diagnosis. Added to the horror that such a diagnosis holds for many people is the additional fear of adverse reactions during treatment.

According to Dr. Hranicky, long-term survivors appear to use some sort of active, engaged strategy for dealing with their disease. She has found that different personalities approach getting well in different ways and that their approach reflects the way they view their illness. Her research shows that this is correlated with their personality structure, and if people stay in distress for a long period of time, they may find that getting well seems difficult. She found that people who found ways to get their psychological needs met positively approached their recovery with more ease. (The psychological needs for each personality type were discussed in detail in Chapter 6.)

Dr. Hranicky uses the Taibi Kahler Stress Profile to help her patients understand their personality strengths, psychological needs, and the distress behaviors they will experience if they do not get their needs met positively. She believes that helping patients design their lifestyle so that they satisfy their psychological needs in positive, constructive, and healthy ways is one of the most important things they can do to regain and maintain their health. She gave several examples that illustrate how she uses the profile.

Patricia is a 58-year-old Reactor who was diagnosed with breast cancer at the age of 22. She had surgery and a widespread bony metastasis. Doctors predicted only a short life expectancy for her. Dr. Hranicky profiled her, and Patricia began developing strategies to get her psychological needs met. She also started following holistic health practices, such as exercise and nutritional management, and setting lifestyle goals. She went back to school and specialized in counseling. She is now in a situation in which she feels accepted and is achieving her need to be successful. She also stopped helping out in a stress-inducing job in the family business. In addition, she moved to an area of the country where she feels more connected to nature and can get her Sensory needs met more easily. She learned to recognize the early warning signs of distress in herself and to take action to get herself out of distress quickly. This has helped Patricia live 15 more years, and she is now in robust health.

According to Dr. Hranicky, when doctors, cancer patients, and their spouses do not communicate, they often get into major conflicts. Frequently this is the result of their different personality structures. The way patients approach recovery may not be what the people around them expect. This can cause major distress in the cancer patient and may make recovery much more difficult. This distress could result in the cancer patient experiencing a phase change, further contributing to the miscommunication.

For example, one of Dr. Hranicky's patients, Mary, experienced a phase change to Promoter. Suddenly she needed more excitement, action, and movement. Her spouse did not understand this shift, as Mary used to be a quiet individual who loved to read, went to the movies, stayed around the house, and played with the dogs. Now she wanted to travel and participate in other exciting activities. Her spouse was confused because it seemed as though he was married to an entirely different person. Mary explained her new psychological needs to her husband so that he understood what was happening. In this way her spouse became an ally in her recovery and not an adversary.

It is important for healthcare providers to explore the stressors in their patients' lives and help them find ways to reduce them. If the providers can do this, the likelihood of their patients living healthier lives greatly improves. Another of Dr. Hranicky's patients, Gary, had prostate cancer at the age of 63. Dr. Hranicky discussed with him his lifestyle and his relationship with his spouse. After a while, Gary explained that he was having an extramarital affair, and the strain of maintaining the secrecy was having serious mental and emotional effects on him. Gary, a Promoter, looked at the negative things he was doing to get his Incident need met and decided he had to find other ways to get this need met positively. Gary loved his exciting life, so finding new and creative ways to get that need met within his marriage was a challenge. He had his wife profiled so that he would understand her needs better. He helped her get her needs met, and she joined him in pursuing the action-oriented and exciting things he wanted to do to get his Incident need met in a positive way. They now are better able to communicate with each other, and Gary says that he has turned his life around for the better. His cancer is in remission.

Dr. Hranicky's research shows that the more successful people are at finding and creating situations that suit their personal success dynamics, the easier it will be for them to generate positive energy, manage stress effectively, maximize their recovery potential, and prevent chronic illness. Unproductive behavior, distress symptoms, or undesirable behavior generally happen when people are not getting their psychological needs met positively. She believes that it is necessary for a care provider to understand the patient's perception of any situation and to recognize the patient's needs. They then can use this knowledge to satisfy the requirements for treating the patient's symptoms successfully. Understanding this information may be one of the most important lifestyle interventions people can use to optimize their health and longevity. She believes that knowing how to connect with other people effectively is one of the most powerful tools healthcare providers have in sustaining transactions that provide energy and rejuvenation.

Dr. Hranicky also believes that healthcare providers should consider the person's environmental preference as an essential part of the diagnostic process in any refined treatment prevention or anti-aging model. She adds that "unhealthy emotions and behaviors that are predictable reflecting chronic distress in a person, can be shifted to more desirable patterns of well-being when individuals are able to connect to the people in their lives that nourish them and 'charge their battery.' "

Placing people in environments in which they are most comfortable means maintaining contact with people who help them get their psychological needs met and with whom they can communicate easily. But environmental preference is more than that. It also means placing them in a work or home environment in which they feel most comfortable. For example, Reactors need to work with or be around groups of close friends. Dreamers prefer to work alone. Workaholics and Persisters prefer working with one other person. Rebels and Promoters want to work with groups of people, but with no strong attachment to the members of the group. They also want freedom to move from group to group. Placing people in an environment in which they are not comfortable is an invitation for them to go into distress.

For example, placing Reactors in an environment in which they have to work alone all day may result in their getting into distress. Similarly, placing Dreamers in an environment in which they have to work closely with groups of people all day may result in their getting into distress. Additionally, having Reactors and Dreamers work together all day is also an invitation for them to go into distress. The Reactor will want to establish a close friendship with the Dreamer. If the Dreamer has not gotten her or his Solitude need met, he or she may feel suffocated and try to push the Reactor away and withdraw from having a friendship. When this happens, the Reactor will feel rejected, and both persons may end up in distress. Chapter 8 explores what each of the six personality types does when in distress. Also explored is what healthcare providers can do proactively to keep patients and staff members from getting into distress, and what they can do retroactively to invite them out of distress when they see the distress behaviors discussed in the next two chapters.

8

Distress

Thus far we have been talking mostly about the positive behaviors of the various personality types. However, when they get into distress, each of the six types has predictable and observable negative behaviors. Many patients are in distress when they visit their doctors or when they enter a hospital. People who are in distress are not capable of clearly hearing what their doctors or nurses are saying to them. Therefore, it is imperative that healthcare professionals know how to invite their patients out of distress so that they hear the message.

Doctors and nurses who can identify the symptoms that indicate their patients are starting to get into distress or are in severe distress can intervene quickly and invite them out of distress. In this way, they will ensure that patients hear their message and are also in a positive frame of mind. It is well documented that patients with a positive attitude recover from illnesses, injuries, and operations much more quickly than those who remain in distress.

This is also true for healthcare administrators. Administrators who can identify the symptoms that indicate their staff members are beginning to get into distress can intervene and invite the staff members out of distress, thereby stopping these individuals' negative behaviors before they disrupt the smooth functioning of the facility. When administrators, doctors, or nurses see the behaviors described in this chapter, they must remember that the people displaying the behaviors are still OK. The behaviors are a cry for help and a warning sign that the person is being mismanaged, is having trouble dealing with something going on in her or his life, or is not getting her or his needs met. In many instances this is what triggers the negative distress behaviors. Understanding this, healthcare professionals may be able to resist more easily the invitation to respond to another person's distress behavior by getting into distress themselves.

In his research, Dr. Kahler identified three levels of distress. These levels include observable and predictable behaviors. According to Dr. Kahler, each of the six personality types may experience stress in a different way, which leads to different responses at each level of distress that are unique to that personality type. His research shows that these levels are sequential; that is, people don't get to the second level of distress without first going through the first level, and they don't get to the third level without initially going through the first and second levels. In keeping with the condominium comparison, described in Chapter 2, Dr. Kahler explains that beneath their personality condominium, people have a doorway (first degree) that leads to a basement (second degree) and ultimately to the cellar of distress (third degree).

Everyone—including doctors, nurses, administrators, staff members, patients, and patients' family members—experiences first-degree distress (the least amount of distress) many times during the day. Usually the distress lasts only a second or two and people return to the positive parts of their personality. However, sometimes individuals experience the distress more severely and descend into their basement. Awareness of the signals that each type exhibits in first-degree distress can help healthcare professionals intervene before major problems ensue.

Second-degree distress is more noticeable and often can result in dysfunctional behavior that frequently ends in people making mistakes, insisting that their way is the only way to do things, and so forth. Some employees attack others around issues of fairness and not being able to think clearly. Others push their ideas and attack people for not being committed to the goals of the team. When people attack others, they invite others to join them in distress. When that happens, some people will make mistakes doing things they usually do very well. Some will shut down. Others will do something to further antagonize the other members of the team, and still others will manipulate, con, lie, and stir up trouble with teammates. When healthcare professionals know the interventions to use to invite each of the six types out of first- and second-degree distress, they can eliminate friction on their management team and improve team cohesiveness and the productivity and profitability of the organization.

When employees of all six types get into third-degree distress, they feel depressed and useless and may appear only to be going through the motions of their jobs. When this happens, they are not capable of thinking clearly and may believe that others care only about themselves. At this point, they frequently stop caring about anything—their job, their appearance, or any activities. This usually happens when they have not gotten their needs met for a prolonged period of time, and probably will require intense intervention to get them out of distress.

What are the warning signs that staff members or patients are getting into distress, and what are the various interventions healthcare providers can use to invite them out of distress so that they can be productive again? The rest of this chapter will answer these questions.

WORKAHOLICS

In first-degree distress, Workaholics expect to be perfect and tend to put off doing things for pleasure until after they finish the job on which they are working. They put off personal pleasure so much that eventually they begin to get into distress about it. They epitomize the old saying, "All work and no play makes Jack a dull boy." All work and no play frequently results in

Workaholics getting into distress. When this happens, Workaholics begin to use big words when little words would do, over-qualify their sentences, and make complicated statements. For example, healthcare professionals might hear a Workaholic in first-degree distress say, "If you want my input, recognizing that all the information is not yet available to me, and recognizing my right to offer, that is to say, provide additional suggestions as I receive, that is, obtain, more information, then as I see it, there are several options, that is, courses of action, available to us." When Workaholics talk like this, they think they are being clearer when they actually are making it very difficult for people to understand them.

To invite people out of first-degree distress, healthcare providers can use the Workaholic's preferred channel and perception to communicate with them. As we saw in Chapter 5, Workaholics' favorite channel is the Requestive channel. Their preferred perception is Thoughts. Therefore, a healthcare provider might say something like, "What do the data show?" Most of the time this simple intervention of channel and perception will result in Workaholics coming out of first-degree distress.

In second-degree distress, Workaholics overcontrol and put on an attacker mask and attack people for not being able to think clearly, for a lack of neatness, for making mistakes, for being late for meetings or missing deadlines, or for not being logical or organized. How can healthcare providers invite a Workaholic out of second-degree distress? When people are in second-degree distress, they are advertising that they are being mismanaged and/or are not getting their needs met positively. Therefore, healthcare professionals should give them a battery charge for the need that corresponds to the behavior they are seeing. As we saw in Chapter 6, the Workaholic's needs are Recognition of Work and Time Structure. Therefore, the healthcare professional can compliment the Workaholic on something he or she has done well—a well-written paper, a good suggestion, a well-handled problem, and so forth. People usually will come out of second-degree distress immediately. However, providers must remember that they cannot make people come out of distress; they can only invite them out. The staff member or patient decides whether to accept the invitation.

Colonel Leslie Newell is a nurse in the Canadian army. She told the following story about a Canadian clinician who had not been trained in pediatrics but frequently was required to treat severely wounded children when on assignment to Afghanistan. Because the clinician was not trained in pediatrics, he was afraid that he could not treat children perfectly and that he would be held responsible for a death that was unavoidable given the extensive nature of the child's injuries. He subsequently sent an e-mail complaining about what was expected of him and stating his frustration.

In his words, he thought it was absolutely irresponsible of anyone to expect him to do his job in Afghanistan and care for the children in a competent and skilled manner when everyone refused to acknowledge the real work that they were doing there and give them the training they needed. He saw himself as a very competent and responsible clinician, but to think that he could function just by taking his adult experience and downsizing it was illogical and incorrect. The thinking was simply faulty, because children are not adults in little-sized bodies. He would not be responsible for this any longer. He announced that he would finish up and then go. He would not go back, because the work was impossible and was killing him.

Colonel Newell is a Workaholic herself and, therefore, understood the problem and knew what she had to do to placate the clinician. However, since she was in Canada, she could only support the doctor through phone calls and e-mail. She tried to give him battery charges by recognizing the work he was doing and by planning together for pediatric training upon his return. She also promised him a better situation. Unfortunately, it was too late. The clinician did not return and, in fact, left the service upon his return to Canada.

The consultant anesthetist at the New Zealand hospital, who was described in Chapter 6, told the story of the husband of one patient who was very upset about his wife's condition. He was very rude, out of control, and verbally attacking staff members. The anesthetist knew the patient's husband was an accountant and could assess from his words, tone, and gestures and from the mask he wore in distress that he was a Workaholic. Therefore, she spoke to him in the Requestive channel and gave him numbers and data. She also told him what an important job he had and gave him a battery charge for Recognition for Work. He calmed down, stopped attacking the staff, was more understanding, and cooperated with the staff.

The anesthetist also was a source of support for members of her staff who were in conflict. She had them role-play the distress areas of the conflict for her and then, based on their personality structures, showed them why they were having conflict. She explained how each preferred to communicate and their motivational needs. They began to look at one another differently and to be more considerate and respectful in their dealings with one another. They are now on good terms, and when they start to miscommunicate, they recall past events and are able to laugh about it. As a result, staff conflict has been greatly reduced.

When people are in distress, they are not capable of thinking clearly. Therefore, if healthcare providers want to talk with people who are in distress, they must first invite them out of distress; if they do not, the people with whom they are interacting will not hear accurately what is being said.

PERSISTERS

In first-degree distress, Persisters focus on what people have done wrong and ignore what they have done right. They expect everyone to be perfect, and believe that they only need to help people correct what they aren't doing right and they will be perfect. After all, they already know how to do the things they are doing right; therefore, there is no need to talk about those things. When speaking, they may use big words and overqualify their sentences. Whereas Workaholics make complicated statements, Persisters ask complicated questions: "Where, exactly, do you want me to stand?" and "What ostensible advantages, that is to say, benefits, does this new program offer us that would supercede or obviate the program that we have been using successfully and reliably, that is to say, profitably, for the past 10 years?"

When healthcare providers hear people talking like this, they can intervene by using the Persister's favorite channel and perception. As we saw in Chapter 5, the Persister's favorite channel is the Requestive channel, and their favorite perception is Opinions. Therefore, healthcare professionals can ask, "What is your opinion?" or "What do you believe we should do?" This usually will result in the Persister stopping his or her first-degree distress behavior and accessing the positive parts of his or her personality.

If healthcare providers do not intervene, the Persister may go into second-degree distress. In second-degree distress, Persisters put on an attacker mask and push their beliefs. They also frequently attack people for a lack of commitment to team goals, quality, values, or morals. For example, healthcare providers might hear a Persister in second-degree distress say something like, "Don't you care what's happening in our hospital?" or "Trust you? Not on your life. You've got the morals of an alley-cat." These are good warning signs that the Persister is not getting her or his needs met. When healthcare providers hear things like this, they can give Persisters a battery charge for their Recognition of Work and Conviction needs. The healthcare provider might say something like, "Ms. Persister, I admire your commitment to providing high-quality healthcare, and I want to thank you for your dedication. I know I can count on you." Most of the time Persisters will accept this invitation and will come out of distress.

Persister doctors and administrators sometimes have difficulty communicating with Reactor nurses or staff members. Dr. Bujold, the North Carolina family practice physician introduced in Chapter 1, has witnessed many circumstances within his own practice and in others where Persister administrators and healthcare providers attempting to drive their organizations forward have been frustrated and angry at staff members for not moving forward with new initiatives. They often expressed their anger by orally attacking staff members. Some of these situations may have been triggered by something as simple as staff members maintaining personal communication with patients rather than electronically documenting phone conversations with patients in accordance with the new electronic health record requirements.

Following these new requirements is important for medical malpractice reasons, and it represents good medical care. However, staff members frequently feel frustrated when attacked and may get into distress about it. Reactors may feel that people in the office do not like them. In these instances, they may get into distress and become ineffective, as we will see shortly. Sometimes staff members feel so hurt that they quit. Patients, especially Reactor patients, like personal attention from staff members and may get upset when staff members with whom they feel comfortable quit. In these instances, patients may leave practices because they have developed better relationships with staff members than with their healthcare providers.

A revolving door of staff members is a very destructive force within a primary care office. Dr. Bujold believes it takes at least two years to fully train a staff member in his office. And now, with all the additional duties healthcare providers are asked to do in regard to quality and safety, it is nearly impossible to accomplish these tasks without a consistent and stable office staff. Dr. Bujold believes he is very fortunate in this regard because some of his employees have worked in his office for more than 20 years.

Dr. John Link, an oncologist who treats more breast cancer patients than any other doctor on the West Coast, is a Reactor in a Workaholic phase. He is a very good doctor, and he always wants to be perfect in his diagnoses and treatment of his patients. Consequently, it was very distressing to him when things did not go as well as he expected. He frequently went into distress, second-guessed himself, and questioned his diagnoses and treatments. After he learned the concepts of Process Communication, he understood himself better and now handles this conflict within himself better. As a result, he is a much better doctor and has a much better bedside manner.

Many of his patients are in distress about their condition. He now understands how different types of patients react when they are in distress, and he is able to deal with them better. Previously, if he made a mistake, he might respond critically to patients and become overcontrolling. This carried over to his home life and was a stressor in his relationships with his wife and his children.

Now, rather than responding to his patients' distress by getting into distress himself, he uses their preferred channel and perception to communicate with them and help them get their needs met as a strategy to invite them out of distress. Once he gets them out of distress, they are able to think clearly and he can communicate with them so that they hear what he is telling them. He also looks at how they are coping with their medical condition. Some patients want a lot of information, so he gives it to them. Other patients get confused if they get a lot of information, so he gives them just enough to satisfy them.

REACTORS

In first-degree distress, Reactors try to please everyone and have a hard time making decisions or asking directly for things. If two people come to a Reactor with contradictory recommendations, a Reactor in first-degree distress may have a hard time deciding what to do. Reactors want everyone to like them, and they frequently put the welfare of others ahead of their own. Instead of asking directly for a day off, Reactors in first-degree distress say things like, "Maybe I could have some time off sometime soon." They also may say "you know" many times in their sentences. How can healthcare providers intervene to invite them out of distress before they get into second-degree distress? As we saw in Chapter 5, the Reactor's favorite channel is the Nurturative channel, and their perception is Emotions. Therefore, healthcare providers may invite them out of distress by saying things like, "How do you feel about this new policy?" or "Will you share your feelings with us about this program?"

In second-degree distress, Reactors put on a drooper mask and make mistakes on things they know how to do very well. They also may laugh at themselves inappropriately, call themselves stupid, or invite people to criticize them. The Reactor's needs are Recognition of Person and Sensory. Therefore, healthcare professionals can invite Reactors out of second-degree distress by giving them a battery charge, for example, "I'm glad you're here" or "I appreciate your concern for our patients." They also can invite Reactors out of distress by talking with them about things Reactors want to talk about. The authors frequently are able to invite Reactors out of second-degree distress by complimenting them on their appearance, on some article of clothing they are wearing, for their concern for others, for their excellent people skills, or for their ability to boost morale in the office. It also is possible to invite them out of distress by spending a few minutes listening to them as they discuss subjects of interest to them.

Reactors in third-degree distress feel depressed, unwanted, and unloved. They frequently withdraw from others and may stop caring about their appearance and their environment.

A Reactor administrator in charge of nurse education at a Kentucky hospital worked with 10 educational activity coordinators. She also had to coordinate her training with doctors. Although she needed the activity coordinators to do things they did not want to do, she did not have any authority to make them do those things. As a result, she was in severe second- and third-degree distress all the time. She felt depressed and withdrew from everyone. She stopped helping her coworkers, stopped socializing with everyone, and ate by herself in her office. She also was making mistakes but was not aware she was making them. She hated telling people they had to do things they did not want to do.

Once she learned the concepts of Process Communication she understood why she was the way she was and realized she was not getting her needs met. Once she understood why she did not like to tell people what to do, she accepted that about herself and gradually developed strategies to get herself out of distress. Initially, she forced herself to interact with her coworkers again. She began to reestablish friendships and got more involved in activities at the hospital. Her job performance improved greatly and, as a result, her relations with her immediate supervisor improved.

DREAMERS

In first-degree distress, Dreamers have difficulty figuring out what to do. If they are asked to do more than one or two things at a time, they feel overwhelmed and may not know which one to do first. They often will begin all of the tasks but not finish any of them. This trait also carries over to their speech. For example, they may start talking about one subject and then shift to an entirely different topic, frequently without finishing the sentence of the first subject. What does this sound like? "Lights are bright . . . Traffic was heavy . . . My wife said that . . . Yesterday my son went . . ." Dreamers in distress also have a tendency to say, "It occurred to me that . . ."

Listening to a Dreamer in first-degree distress can be painful for the other five types if Dreamer is not a well-developed part of the other person's personality structure. Workaholics want information in a logical sequence and may think the Dreamers are wasting time. Persisters want the important information and quickly may lose patience. Reactors may feel sorry for the Dreamers and want to console them. Rebels won't be having any fun listening and probably will tune the speaker out. Promoters want the bottom line and may walk away. This is one reason Dreamers often are not called on to contribute to discussions. Because they volunteer their ideas only when invited, their insights frequently are lost to the team.

How can healthcare providers invite Dreamers out of first-degree distress? Again, the answer is to use their favorite channel and perception. The channel to use with a Dreamer is the Directive channel and the perception is Inaction. Leaders can say something like, "Tell me one thing you are going to do today to improve patient safety here in the hospital." Obviously, healthcare providers must tailor their speech to what the Dreamer is talking about. For example, if a Dreamer is talking about a project, an administrator might say something like, "Tell me one thing you did on the project" or "Tell me one thing you are going to do today to advance the project."

What do Dreamers do in second-degree distress? They shut down and do nothing until someone tells them to do something. Ryan Kopper, the adventure recreation facilitator introduced in Chapter 6, was running an adventure course with Dreamer, Reactor, and Rebel inpatients one Saturday. This was usually a difficult group because the Dreamers and Reactors did not enjoy doing the activity and usually went into distress during the program. The Dreamers shut down and barely participated, and the Reactors frequently made mistakes. The Rebels liked the activity but didn't always follow directions and often clowned around.

Kopper decided he had to modify the way he taught the course if he was going to keep the inpatients out of distress. After a period of time, he stopped the activity and gave the Dreamers an opportunity to reflect on what they had done and what it meant. He also allowed them to go off by themselves so they could get their Solitude need met. The adventure program lasted two and a half hours. During that time, the Dreamers got about 45 minutes of solitude interspersed throughout the session.

He spoke to the Reactors in the Nurturative channel and gave them opportunities to tell everyone how they felt about what they were doing. Periodically he ran fun games that the Rebels liked doing and gave them a chance to tell everyone what they liked and didn't like about the games. In this way, everyone's needs were met. The Dreamers got their Solitude need met. The Reactors got their Recognition of Person need met by being able to socialize and use their interpersonal skills, and the Rebels had so much fun throughout the program that they were grinning from ear to ear the entire time. There were no behavior problems during the entire session.

The staff members were surprised that there were no behavior problems. Therefore, Kopper conducted a debrief of the exercise to explain what he had done and the reasons for it. The other staff members noted that usually there was a power struggle when these patients were on the adventure course, but that day there were none. He asked their opinions about why there were no power struggles that day. He also asked what usually happens when they tell a Rebel what to do. The staff replied that the Rebels refuse to do it, adding that it happens all the time. Kopper explained what he had done to help the patients get their needs met, and he suggested things the other staff members could do when working with these patients.

REBELS

In first-degree distress, Rebels may act stupid, get impatient, disrupt meetings to attract attention, socialize with others off-topic, make inappropriate statements to irritate other team members, or not give people enough information to do the task they have been assigned. In acting stupid, they may say things in a whiny voice like, "This is hard," "I don't get it," or "I can't."

How can healthcare providers invite Rebels out of first-degree distress? The Rebels' favorite channel is the Emotive channel, and their perception is Reactions, that is, likes and dislikes. Therefore, healthcare professionals can say things like, "Hey, what did you like about the meeting today?" or "What don't you like about this new project?" In most instances, Rebels will accept this invitation and come out of first-degree distress. Why do administrators, doctors, and nurses want to know what Rebels don't like? Because once Rebels tell people what they don't like, they forget about it. Until then, it may fester in them like an open sore and may result in their going into second-degree distress.

What do Rebels do in second-degree distress? They blame others, become stubborn, insist on their own way, disrupt meetings, and may sabotage a project with an "I'll show you" attitude in order to get revenge. How can healthcare providers invite Rebels out of second-degree distress? They can help them get their needs met for Playful Contact by sharing a joke with them, speaking to them in an upbeat and energetic way, providing opportunities for them to use their creativity, allowing time during the day when they can have some fun, singing with them, allowing Rebel employees to have fun things in their office, and allowing them to move around throughout the day.

Jan Lee is the CEO of PaceLine Communication Solutions. She is a Rebel and was going into the hospital to have an operation. She told the nurses she wanted the operation to be fast, fun, and easy. They laughed and she kept telling jokes as they prepared her for the operation. The surgeon came in to the room to talk with her prior to the operation. He entered wearing a blanket draped over his shoulder like a superhero cape. Lee told him he looked like a superhero and he immediately replied, "I am a superhero and I am here to take your order." He immediately established a bond with Lee, who laughed, relaxed, and was confident that the operation would go well. Another doctor on the team was a Workaholic, and Lee gave him a battery charge for Recognition of Work. A third doctor on the team was a Reactor in a Workaholic phase. She gave him battery charges for Recognition for Work and Recognition of Person. The operation went very well.

PROMOTERS

In first-degree distress, Promoters expect others to fend for themselves, and they do not aid people who may need their support. "I'm going to make a man out of you if I have to break you in two trying," "Not tough enough, huh," and "If you can't stand the heat, get out of the kitchen" are sayings that exemplify the spirit of first-degree Promoter distress. Promoters in first-degree distress also frequently say "you" when referring to themselves. For example, "When you're making a report to the board of directors and you have a lot of bad news to give them and you are afraid they may want to exercise more control, then you have a decision to make—tell the truth and let the chips fall where they may or gloss over some of the bad news." What the Promoter really is saying here is, "When I am making a report to the board of directors and I have a lot of bad news to give them . . .”

How can healthcare professionals invite Promoters out of first-degree distress? The Promoter's favorite channel is the Directive channel, and their perception is Action. Therefore, leaders can say to them, “Tell me what you did when that happened to you” or “Tell me what you are going to do.” Most of the time, Promoters will accept this invitation and will come out of first-degree distress.

What do Promoters do in second-degree distress? They put on a blamer mask and manipulate, con, make fools of others, set up fights or arguments between team members, tell lies about team members, engage in negative competition, and find ways to turn the tables on those they blame for things that have happened to them.

Ryan Kopper, who was mentioned earlier, one day saw a 15-year-old female Promoter patient running across the campus. He assumed she was going AWOL from the institution and ran after her. As he neared her, he used the Directive channel and told her to stop. She did. He then told her to listen to him, adding that if she did not like what he had to say, she could continue running. She told him she had wanted to make a phone call but the counselor would not let her. He pointed out that she was running in the wrong direction and told her where the nearest phone was. As they walked toward the phone, he told her to tell him why the counselor would not let her make a phone call. She replied that she refused to do something they wanted her to do, so, as a consequence, she was not allowed to make a phone call. A power struggle ensued between her and the staff and she fled. Because the staff was not able to work with her, Kopper negotiated a deal with her. He would let her make the phone call if she then did what the staff wanted her to do. She agreed, made her phone call, and did what the staff wanted her to do.

After the incident, Kopper explained to the staff what he had done and the reasons for it. He explained that the girl was a Promoter, that her need was Incidence, and that if she did not get the need met positively, she would become obstinate in an effort to get the need met negatively. He suggested some things the staff members could do to help the girl get her needs met positively, and from then on the relationship between the staff members and the girl improved dramatically.

In another instance, a patient in a hospital was about to have an operation on his shoulder. The anesthesiologist came in and began to explain what was going to happen. As he was finishing, another anesthesiologist came in and very arrogantly dismissed the first anesthesiologist. He continued to talk to the patient dismissively. The patient had asked to be kept awake during the operation so that he could see what was going on. However, a drape was placed in front of the patient's face. He asked that the drape be removed so that he could see what they were doing. The anesthesiologist objected, but the patient insisted and the drape was removed. During the operation the anesthesiologist made comments that the patient thought were uncalled for, and at one point the anesthesiologist told the surgeon that he should do something one way. The patient objected and told them what he wanted them to do. Finally the surgeon told the anesthesiologist that he would do what the patient wanted.

Later, the patient told the surgeon that if he had to have another operation in the future, he did not want the anesthesiologist on his team. He added that if the anesthesiologist was on the operating team, he would leave rather than go through with the operation. The doctor was surprised and asked why he felt that way. The patient recounted what had happened and told the surgeon some of the comments the anesthesiologist made during the operation. The doctor had not heard the comments, as he was concentrating on the operation. Why was the anesthesiologist in so much distress? The patient believes a contributing factor was that, at the time of the surgery, the anesthesiologist's leg was in a cast and he was in considerable pain. That's the point. When people display the negative behaviors described in this chapter, there is a reason for it. Healthcare professionals have to remember that the person is OK; it is the behavior that is wrong. If healthcare providers remember this, it will be easier for them to keep themselves from getting into distress, and they will be more able to invite others out.

What happens in third-degree distress? At this level, all six personality types put on a despairer mask and feel unloved, unwanted, and depressed. Workaholics reject others for not thinking clearly; Persisters cease to be team players and quit; Reactors stop caring about their appearance, their jobs, or their families; Dreamers shut down; Rebels find creative ways to get even; and Promoters abandon others. How can healthcare providers invite people out of third-degree distress? By helping them get their psychological needs met positively. Most of the time, people will accept the invitation and will come out of distress. However, if they are in third-degree distress, they probably have been in distress for some time and will not have enough energy to stay out of distress for any length of time. Keeping them out of distress probably will require enhanced interventions.

The next chapter looks at what healthcare providers do when in distress, and what they can do to keep themselves from getting into distress.

9

Healthcare Providers in Distress

W hat do healthcare providers do when in distress, and what can their colleagues, supervisors, and others do to invite them out of distress to improve their performance and job satisfaction, and patient safety and satisfaction?

Colonel Leslie Newell, the Canadian army nurse introduced in Chapter 8, is a Workaholic. She tells the following story about her own distress when other people were given credit for work that she had done. Colonel Newell was working in Bosnia as part of a Canadian medical team. A five-year-old girl named Irma was playing in the street outside a store while a playmate and her mother were shopping inside. A mortar round exploded in the store and Irma was seriously injured. She was taken to a Sarajevo hospital, but because of a shortage of medical supplies, there was not much the doctors could do. It was clear that Irma had to be evacuated if they were to have any chance of saving her life. Colonel Newell planned and prepared for Irma's evacuation while authorities tried for several days to negotiate Irma's release. Each day, Irma's condition worsened and her chances for survival lessened. Eventually Colonel Newell and a medical technician named Laurie evacuated Irma to Ancona, Italy. A British trauma team then flew to Ancona and took Irma and her father and sister to London.

Two years later, Colonel Newell returned to Ancona while en route to Rwanda. In the Operations Center at the airfield she saw a very beautiful print of a painting that had been commissioned by the British as a fundraiser for Operation Irma. For $50, people could be part of the legacy of the rescue. The print was signed by every member of the rescue team with an enclosed narrative text crediting a British medical team for her evacuation from Sarajevo to Ancona and onward to London.

At that point, Colonel Newell realized that her work and efforts had been erased from time because someone else had taken credit for the evacuation by the Canadian team. Every member of the crew that had rescued Irma—except Colonel Newell and her medical technician, Laurie—had signed the print. When Colonel Newell saw that her and Laurie's efforts had not been recorded accurately, she went into severe distress—not because she wanted to be known as a hero, but because, as a Workaholic, she needed their work to be acknowledged and accurately depicted in the narrative. This affected her deeply and, until she was able to get others to recognize the work she currently was doing, she was not as effective as she normally had been. Workaholics do not value self-generated recognition for their work. On the contrary, they discount it.

Before going further, let's analyze the distress behaviors in the story in Chapter 1 about Elaine Bromiley, the patient who died during an attempted operation. The following account is taken from the article "Have You Ever Made a Mistake?"[21] The author is Martin Bromiley, the husband of Elaine Bromiley. He attended the postsurgery hearing in which the case was discussed.

According to the article, Elaine Bromiley was scheduled to have endoscopic sinus surgery and a septoplasty in March 2005. Everyone on the operating team was very experienced, very skilled, and well respected. A very thorough pre-op assessment was carried out, and there were no significant concerns. The proposed anesthetic technique was to avoid tracheal intubation and maintain the airway with a laryngeal mask. There was no pre-oxygenation.

Anesthesia was induced, but it was not possible to insert the flexible laryngeal mask due to increased tone in the jaw muscles. The consultant anesthetist tried two sizes of laryngeal mask but could not insert either. The patient's oxygen saturation dropped to 40%, and the anesthetists attempted to ventilate the lungs with 100% oxygen using a facemask and oral airway but were unsuccessful. The anesthetist decided to try tracheal intubation to overcome the problems with the airway. Another anesthetist consultant and the ENT (ear, nose, and throat) surgeon joined the group and made further unsuccessful attempts at laryngoscopy. Meanwhile, a nurse left the operating room and arranged a bed in intensive care. She returned and announced that a bed was available. The anesthetists looked at her as if to say she was overreacting. Another nurse asked a colleague to get the "trachy machine." On her return she announced to the consultants that the tracheotomy set was available. They ignored her and continued to attempt laryngoscopy and intubation. Finally, after 35 minutes they decided to abandon the procedure and allow the patient to wake up.

Once the anesthetist consultant was satisfied that the patient was breathing satisfactorily, she was transferred to the recovery room. The nurses in the recovery room were not happy with her condition and transferred her to intensive care. She never regained consciousness. She went into a coma and died 13 days later.

Let's look at this case from a Process Communication point of view. We can conclude that both anesthetists were Persisters in distress. When in distress, people are not capable of thinking clearly. As we saw in the previous chapter, Persisters in distress know that they are right and continue doing what they are doing. Frequently, when they are in distress, they do not listen to suggestions from other people. Indeed, they may not even hear what others are saying. It is not clear what personality type the nurses were, but they may have been Reactors. In distress, Reactors want to please everyone and often remain quiet rather than risk antagonizing another person. As a result, a patient died.

What could the nurses or someone on the operating team have done to get the anesthetist consultant out of distress? They might have used his preferred channel and perception and given him a battery charge for Recognition of Work. What might this sound like? "Dr. A, you are an outstanding anesthetist and you have participated in many operations. In your opinion, should we consider getting the trachy machine?" Healthcare professionals need to remember that they cannot make people come out of distress; they only can invite them out. It is up to the individual to decide whether to accept the invitation. Therefore, it is possible that the anesthetist consultant may not have stopped to think about other possible approaches. However, it is almost certain that he would continue his distress behavior without a battery charge for his psychological needs.

At the postsurgery review, the consultants said they knew what they should have done but were not sure why they did not do it. From a Process Communication point of view, the reason they did not do it is because people in distress are not able to think clearly. Healthcare professionals must keep themselves out of distress by getting their needs met every day. When they see colleagues in distress they can invite them out by helping them get their motivational needs met positively. If they do this, they can greatly reduce the number of medical errors in their facility.

To give you an opportunity to test your ability to implement the concepts of Process Communication when dealing with people in distress, several true stories describing healthcare providers in distress have been included. Following each story are a few questions that ask what you would do in this situation. After that is a summary of what the healthcare provider in that actual situation said and did and the results. Also included is a list of suggestions for healthcare providers to help them get their psychological needs met positively so they keep themselves out of distress.

STORY ONE

Dr. Mark Weinert, an anesthetist in Germany, told the story of a brilliant surgeon who frequently chastised other members of the surgical team for not moving fast enough during operations. The surgeon was overly dramatic and used the Directive channel to order team members to do things. He manipulated members of the surgical team, which led to constant crises in the operating room. Because of his attitude, the nurses were afraid of him and frequently made mistakes when he shouted at them. For example, they sometimes handed him the wrong instruments. When this happened, he would fly into a rage and throw the instruments back at them. As a result, no one wanted to work with him. During one emergency operation he grew impatient with the surgical team and began criticizing them.

TEST YOUR UNDERSTANDING OF THE CONCEPTS

What is the surgeon's personality type?

_____

What is his motivational need?

_____

(Continued)

What is his favorite channel and perception?

_____

What would you do?

_____

What would you say?

_____

What Dr. Weinert Did

Dr. Weinert knew that the surgeon was a Promoter who needed to be doing something. Therefore, Weinert used the Directive channel and told the surgeon to put an arterial line in the patient. Normally Dr. Weinert did this himself, but he wanted to keep the surgeon busy so that he would allow the other team members to do their work. The surgeon did as he was told. Once he started doing something, he stopped criticizing the other team members and they were able to communicate with him. In another emergency, Dr. Weinert had the surgeon perform CPR on a patient. This gave him something important to do and also got him out of the way so the other team members could do their jobs. After the operation, Dr. Weinert thanked the surgeon for saving the patient's life. The surgeon was happy because he played an important role in the operation and also because everyone gave him credit for saving the patient's life. From then on, he stopped criticizing the other members of the surgical team and was calmer and more patient. There is no clear thinking occurring when people are in distress. (See Figure 9.1 for some suggestions of ways to help people get their Incident needs met positively.)

Need: Incidence

Promoters have a need for excitement and thrills so that they don't become bored, restless, or agitated. They also like challenges, risks, and competition—short term goals with quick results or large payoffs. They live on the edge and need to be active in their lives. You can help them get their need for incidence met by helping them set up personal or professional challenges, engage in new projects that are risky yet do not threaten their well-being. They also can get their needs met by involving themselves with exciting, action-oriented people. Here are some suggestions of ways you can help them get their Incident need met.

- Assign them exciting projects.
- Provide quick rewards for successes or improved performance.
- Find ways to help them look good to their peers or supervisors.
- Ensure that they get involved in active or exciting projects, so that work time is not dull or routine.
- Brainstorm with them about ways processes can be done better.
- Assign them a leadership role in devising ways to improve processes.
- Have them work on projects that give quick recognition or rewards.

Figure 9.1 Promoter action plan.
Source: Copyright © 1997 Taibi Kahler Associates.

STORY TWO

Dr. Weinert told another story about a nurse in the operating room who assisted the anesthetist during operations. The nurse frequently made mistakes and was absolutely of no use during emergencies. Whenever members of the operating team needed something in a hurry and told the nurse to get it, the nurse gave them something entirely different. Other team members raised concerns about the safety of their patients, and several of the anesthetists wanted the nurse fired.

TEST YOUR UNDERSTANDING OF THE CONCEPTS

What is the personality type of the nurse?

_____

What are his psychological needs?

_____

What is his favorite channel and perception?

_____

What would you do?

_____

What would you say?

_____

What Dr. Weinert Did

Dr. Weinert realized the nurse was a Reactor in distress. Therefore, he began to greet the nurse by name when he came to the operating theater and told him he was glad he was there. He also began spending a few minutes talking with the nurse and listened carefully to what he was saying. One day the nurse showed Dr. Weinert a new tattoo he had on his shoulder. It was a picture of his mother, who had died recently. Dr. Weinert commented on what a sweet idea that was and added that the nurse must have had a very close relationship with his mother.

The Results

The nurse's work performance changed completely. He stopped making mistakes and became a very valuable member of the operating team, even in emergencies. Now, when team members ask for something, he gives them what they asked for. Other members of the operating team noted the improvement and also began to call him by his first name. At a social event, the nurse told Dr. Weinert how happy he was to be at the hospital. He said that he previously had worked at private hospitals in Australia and people either didn't address him at all or called him by his surname. He was miserable and changed hospitals. No one in the department talks about getting him fired now. (See Figure 9.2 for

---

Needs: Recognition of Person and Sensory

Reactors need to be recognized as a special and unique person. Personal relationships are important to them, both at home and in their professional life. They need to be around people who like them and care about them and with whom they show warmth and caring. They will work best as part of a team in which they feel accepted, wanted and noticed as an individual. Here are some ways to help them meet this need for Personal Attention and Appreciation:

- Be cordial when possible and make eye contact with them.
- Greet them with a smile whenever you see them and call them by name.
- Ask them about their families—be authentic.
- Celebrate their accomplishments with parties and social recognition.
- Sing Happy Birthday to them on their birthdays.
- Allow them to arrange their workspace in an attractive manner.
- Allow them to keep flowers or plants around their workspace, if possible.
- Encourage them to wear soft and comfortable, albeit appropriate, clothes and shoes whenever possible.
- Encourage them to seek out and make good friends at work.
- Encourage them to keep photographs of loved ones where they can see them often.
- Have them work with people who appreciate their personality.
- Encourage them to participate in the social activities in the facility.

Figure 9.2 Reactor action plan.
Source: Copyright © 1997 Taibi Kahler Associates.

a few suggestions of ways to help people get their Recognition of Person and Sensory needs met positively.)

STORY THREE

The clinical practice manager at a large multipractice group in the Midwest found that communicating with physicians on a daily basis can be a tricky proposition for even the most seasoned healthcare managers. He had worked in healthcare for more than 10 years, 3 of them in management, and considered himself adequately prepared to handle the ins and outs of physician communication. After completing training in Process Communication, he realized just how unprepared he actually was. His biggest aha in the training was the concept of focusing more on the person's needs and less on the content of the discussion. Once he was able to recognize the signs of distress and then speak that person's language, communicating with physicians and other managers suddenly became exponentially more efficient. Business decisions and conflict resolution that used to take weeks to move on began happening in days.

To illustrate this, the clinical practice manager told the following story about an incident regarding physician scheduling on a holiday weekend.

The Story

"One of the full-time physicians who regularly covers in our practice had been working 50+ hours a week for a couple of months. By choice, she decided to work weekends in addition to her regular schedule. When it came time to set the schedule for May, she informed me she was going to scale back her weekends and spend more time at home. As the schedule started filling in, I grew concerned about the holiday weekend because we had little to no coverage in a very busy practice. At first, she was reluctant to work any that weekend. Understanding the psychological needs of her personality type, I was able to communicate with her using her preferred channel of communication and we eventually agreed that she would help cover the Saturday shift if I agreed to leave her off the Sunday schedule. I was able to cover the Sunday shifts with other physicians, and we went into the weekend fully staffed. I was headed out of town with my family, expecting the weekend to operate as we planned. On my way home Sunday morning, I took a call from our office stating we were short a physician. In my haste to get out of town I forgot to call one of the residents covering Sunday. The resident was planning on coming in at 3:00 instead of 12:00 as I had thought. I told my staff to continue seeing patients while I worked on a solution. I frantically began calling other physicians to see if any of them could come in until 3:00, and after about five or six calls, I finally found one who was willing to come in. When he showed up, though, the physician I had promised would be off was already there. My staff, unbeknownst to me, had called her before calling me and left her a message. She came in not knowing I already had covered the shift with someone else. She stayed and worked until 3:00, and the physician I contacted left.

"I fully expected to receive a verbal lashing of some sort the next working day. To no surprise on my part, she had e-mailed (3 paragraphs and 500 words later) the department head and my boss (who went through Process Communication training with me). Needless to say, she was quite upset we had wasted her time, and I neglected to honor my promise to her. Her e-mail was laced with critical observations about what I did wrong and how I failed to value her time. She demanded assurances that I would never make a mistake of this magnitude again, and she requested my plan of action for months to come. She was in full-blown attack mode, and I was her target."

TEST YOUR UNDERSTANDING OF THE CONCEPTS

What is the personality type of the angry doctor?

_____

What are the psychological needs of this personality type?

_____

What is her favorite channel and perception?

_____

What are you going to do?

_____

What are you going to say to her?

_____

What the Clinical Practice Manager Did

"Prior to the Process Communication training, I most likely would have been sucked into the vortex of distress. I have a Workaholic base, so my natural defense would have been to come back at her with the logic and reasoning behind my mistake. We probably would have spent several days saying things we didn't really mean, going back and forth with each other about the facts of the situation and getting absolutely nowhere close to a resolution. Our relationship would have been strained simply because neither one of us could manage to get out of distress long enough to ignore the content of our conversation. Eventually we would have come to a conclusion and there would have been plenty of residual baggage carried over to the next time something like this occurred.

"As a result of the Process Communication training, I now know there is a better way. I sent a three-sentence-long e-mail to her Sunday night. In the first sentence I gave her a battery charge for her Persister Conviction need. I immediately thanked her for the dedication and commitment she showed to the organization and apologized for wasting her time. The second sentence shifted the blame entirely on me. I didn't waste time discussing facts or the circumstances surrounding the error; I simply accepted the blame and acknowledged that I had failed to uphold my end of the deal. These first two sentences were my attempt at inviting her out of second-degree distress. The third sentence was another battery charge and another invitation to come out of distress.

The Result

"When I came into the office Tuesday morning, a few of the other physicians who were aware of what happened spent a few minutes joking with me about it and warning me about the impending rampage when the doctor showed up. (She has a reputation for blowing up when things go wrong.) When she came in and after she got settled, I walked up to her and essentially reiterated what my e-mail said. I acknowledged her commitment and dedication to the department and put the blame entirely on me. Her reply was, 'That's okay. I know it wasn't done intentionally. How was your vacation?' I was stunned at the turnaround. We have gone through four such schedule rotations since then, including two with holidays, and she has not mentioned my error even once." (See Figure 9.3 for some suggestions of ways to help people get their Conviction and Recognition of Work needs met positively.)

Need: Conviction and Recognition of Work

It is important for Persisters to lead a life consistent with their beliefs, values and opinions. Whenever possible they like to exercise their influence, impacting upon the growth and direction of others. They need to be around others who share their high standards of integrity, dependability, and trust. You can help them get their needs met in the following ways:

- Ask their opinions of ways to improve patient safety and satisfaction.
- Give them positive feedback on the quality of their work.
- Reaffirm daily to them the value of their accomplishments.
- Reward them for their dedicated service.
- Encourage them to prioritize every day what they believe will be the best investment of their time and energy to ensure quality of effort.
- Involve them in meaningful projects to improve the systems at the facility.
- Encourage them to join important committees at the healthcare facility.
- Have them speak to local groups about healthcare matters.
- Suggest they write articles about things they believe in.

Figure 9.3 Persister action plan.
Source: Copyright © 1997 Taibi Kahler Associates.

STORY FOUR

Dr. Weinert told the authors the following story. One of the anesthetists in his hospital in New Zealand is a cardiac and pediatric specialist. Whenever they operated on a sick child, everything had to be perfect or the specialist would attack the nurses and others. When attacked, the Reactor nurses often cried, went into distress, and made mistakes. During a cardiac bypass operation it is necessary to unplug the ultrasound probe at a certain point in the operation or the patient can get burned. The anesthetist always anticipated when it would be necessary to unplug the probe, and before Dr. Weinert could unplug it, the anesthetist would tell him, "We need to unplug."

Dr. Weinert is a Workaholic and used to respond by going into distress because he thought the anesthetist thought he was stupid. In dealing with the nurses, the anesthetist continually focused on the one thing that was not good enough. If he could not find something to criticize, he disconnected something and pointed out that it was not connected. One day when he could not find anything to criticize, he took saline solution, washed away the ink on a medical document, and said, "This is a medical document. You are not using a true pen."

TEST YOUR KNOWLEDGE OF THE CONCEPTS

What is the anesthetist's personality type?

_____

What are his psychological needs?

_____

What is his favorite channel and perception?

_____

What would you do?

_____

What would you say?

_____

What Dr. Weinert Did

After learning the concepts of Process Communication, Dr. Weinert realized that the specialist was a Persister in distress. He realized it was important to the anesthetist that everything go well. Thus he understood that the anesthetist was not telling him he was stupid; he just wanted to make certain the patient was going to be OK. Dr. Weinert began to compliment the anesthetist on his accomplishments and especially on his conviction for, and commitment to, the safety of his patients. Dr. Weinert also began to ask him his opinion of various medical issues and to help contribute to his medical education. Specifically he asked him, "What can you teach me today?" The anesthetist stopped attacking him and the nurses, and they began to function as a more effective team. For this strategy to be effective, the compliments must be sincere and as specific as possible. Generalizations are not nearly so effective as specific compliments.

STORY FIVE

A nurse consultant in charge of nurse education at a North Carolina hospital had a supervisor who was in a lot of distress because things were not going well at the hospital. The hospital was up for Continuing Medical Education reaccreditation, and it had let so many administrative things slide that many people did not think it would get accredited. As a result, relations between the nurse and her supervisor were strained. As the date for reaccreditation drew nearer, the distress level of the nurse's boss increased. She attacked the nurse almost daily and criticized everything she was doing.

TEST YOUR UNDERSTANDING OF THE CONCEPTS

What is the personality type of the nurse's boss?

_____

What are the needs of this personality type?

_____

What is the boss's favorite channel and perception?

_____

What would you do?

_____

What would you say?

_____

What the Nurse Did

Previously the nurse would have responded by going into distress herself. Instead, she continued to speak to her boss in the Requestive channel and to give her battery charges for her commitment and her accomplishments. Her boss's distress level decreased. In an effort to improve the relationship, the nurse began asking her boss for guidance. She would explain a problem to her boss, tell her how she planned to deal with it, and ask her opinion of the proposed solution. She also began to compliment her boss for things the boss did that worked out well. As a result, her relationship with her supervisor gradually improved. The supervisor stopped attacking her and became much more supportive.

STORY SIX

When Major General (ret.) Gale Pollock, former acting surgeon general of the Army Medical Department, was a lieutenant colonel, she took over a dysfunctional department at an army medical center. One of the experienced members on her staff was uncooperative, moody, and a chronic complainer about the workplace. He was faultless and blamed everyone else for everything that happened. He often said things like, "Yes, but that won't work around here." General Pollock knew she had to do something quickly to invite him out of distress, as it is difficult to motivate new staff when their first encounter with experienced staff members is filled with complaints.

TEST YOUR UNDERSTANDING OF THE CONCEPTS

What is the experienced staff member's personality type?

_____

What is the psychological need of that type?

_____

What is the favorite channel and perception of that type?

_____

What would you do?

_____

What would you say to him?

_____

What General Pollock Did

General Pollock realized that the staff member was a Rebel and that something had happened that was bothering him. She stopped him in the hall one day and asked about it. He replied that he wanted to wear an operating room cap that his wife had made for him, but the leadership of the operating room would not let him. She told him that if he would put on a disposable hat over his own as he entered the operating room hallway and then remove the disposable one as he exited the hallway, there was no reason he could not wear his own hat anywhere else in the hospital. He told her that "they" would not let him. She assured him that she would support him and told him to tell her if anyone harassed him about it. Such a little thing, but it turned him into a huge advocate for General Pollock's department. (See Figure 9.4 for some

---

Need: Playful Contact

Rebels thrive on external stimulation. They dislike routine and simplicity so they need to be able to move around physically, move in and out of various situations and make contact with different people. They also need an environment with brightly colored lights, loud music, bright colors, and mechanical gadgets and they like people who are fun and exciting to be around. Rebels work best when they keep themselves charged up with lots of external stimulation. You can help them get their needs met by:

- Being light hearted with them.
- Speaking to them in an upbeat tone.
- Encouraging their creativity.
- Suggesting that they participate in fun activities at the healthcare facility.
- To the extent possible, allowing them to individualize the way they decorate their workspace.
- Letting them listen to music periodically during the workday.
- Suggesting they use breaks and their lunch hour to move around and visit with others.
- Encouraging them to take brief exercise and stretch breaks throughout the day.
- Having them attend professional conferences.

Figure 9.4 Rebel action plan.

Source: Copyright © 1997 Taibi Kahler Associates.

suggestions of ways to help people get their Playful Contact need met positively.)

STORY SEVEN

Another member of General Pollock's staff was the informal leader of the department. He consistently worked to oppose any action or recommendations by the leadership. He disagreed with every policy change and every new directive that was issued. He then went to the other doctors one at a time and convinced them that the new directives and policies were stupid. He got them to agree that none of them would follow the new policies or implement the new directives. He attacked people who did not agree with him, often shouting at them. In general, he intimidated everyone and usually got his way.

TEST YOUR UNDERSTANDING OF THE CONCEPTS

What is the personality type of the staff member?

What are the psychological needs of the staff member?

What is his favorite channel and perception?

What would you do?

_____

What would you say?

_____

What General Pollock Did

General Pollock assessed the staff member as a Persister. She asked him his opinions of possible courses of action and listened to the reasons he thought his suggested courses of action were important. She did not have to agree with him or do things the way he believed they should be done. She only had to spend a few moments listening to him and asking for clarification. He almost immediately stopped being the source of many problems in the department—an example of a few minutes invested for a huge return.

STORY EIGHT

The anesthetist consultant from New Zealand, who was introduced in Chapter 6, constantly clashed with a colleague with whom she had worked for many years. He was in considerable distress. He wanted everything to be perfect, and he kept finding fault with everything she did. He constantly attacked her for not being serious and for not doing things the way he thought they should be done. As a result, she was not able to connect with him. Because she is a Rebel, her favorite channel is the Emotive channel; however, her colleague was not open to it. This resulted in constant miscommunication and misunderstanding.

**TEST YOUR UNDERSTANDING
OF THE CONCEPTS**

What is the personality type of the anesthetist's colleague?

_____

What are his psychological needs?

_____

What is his favorite channel and perception?

_____

What would you do?

_____

What would you say to him?

_____

What the Anesthetist Did

The anesthetist believed her colleague was a Persister in a Workaholic phase. Therefore, she began to deal with him in the Requestive channel and to give him information and data. She also gave him battery charges by recognizing the excellent work he was doing. In addition, she began to ask his opinion of things. Their entire relationship changed. He stopped attacking her and began to respect her and to appreciate the job she was doing. Her life at work greatly improved.
(See Figure 9.5 for some suggestions of ways to help people get their Recognition of Work and Time Structure needs met positively.)

Needs: Recognition for Work and Time Structure

Workaholics take pride in their ability to think and perform and they are willing to work hard to reach their goals. They prefer to set their own goals but can also work as a team player to accomplish something they accept as worthwhile. Achievement is important to them and you can help them get this need met by praising them for their hard work and their good work. For example:

- Recognize their accomplishments every day.
- Compliment them on their hard work.
- Reward them for jobs accomplished.
- Encourage them to display certificates, plaques, or awards they have received.
- Have them make lists and cross items off as they complete them.
- Have them set short, medium and long term goals and check their progress regularly.
- Encourage them to take time each day to set priorities and focus on doing what is most important.
- Don't assign them so much to do that they cannot do everything well.
- Tell them to be frank and honest about what they can and cannot do.
- Give them advance notice of meetings and compliment them when they are on time.
- Start and end meetings on time.

Figure 9.5 Workaholic action plan.
Source: Copyright © 1997 Taibi Kahler Associates.

STORY NINE

The doctor in charge of the residency program in the family medicine department at a hospital in Hawaii, who was introduced in Chapter 1, told the authors that one of the residents in the program was overwhelmed with the number of tasks he had to deal with every day. He seemed unable to prioritize them and he shut down. As a result, he was not completing any of the tasks required of him.

TEST YOUR UNDERSTANDING OF THE CONCEPTS

What is the resident's personality type?

_____

What is the resident's psychological need?

_____

What is his favorite channel and perception?

_____

What would you do?

_____

What would you say?

_____

What the Director Did

The director realized the resident was a Dreamer and needed solitude and direction. Therefore, using the Directive channel and the perception of Inaction, the director helped the resident prioritize his tasks. He told the resident to focus on one task, and after completing it, move to the next task on his list. He also told him to make certain he took a few minutes to be by himself several times a day so that he got his Solitude need met. In addition, he told him to refer to the action plan in the personality profile booklet he had given him and make certain he did some of those things daily to ensure he got his psychological needs met positively every day.

Some people may believe that they should not have to help adults prioritize the things they have to do. However, the

---

Need: Solitude

Dreamers need alone time, where they can spend time by themselves, undisturbed by people, noises, or outside demands. When they meet their need for Solitude, they feel better, work more productively, and are able to reflect on their life and their goals. Here are some examples of how you can help Dreamers satisfy this need.

- Ensure they have some alone time 3 or 4 times each day without any interruptions.
- Suggest they brown bag their lunch occasionally and eat by themselves.
- Encourage them to spend a few minutes alone at the beginning and end of each workday.
- Encourage them to set aside time to read journals or magazine articles that are relevant to their field.
- Suggest they plan regular times each day when they can work alone and not be disturbed.
- Allow them time to take a walk alone during lunch or before or after work.

Figure 9.6 Dreamer action plan.
Source: Copyright © 1997 Taibi Kahler Associates.

director has learned that people must be dealt with individually to tap fully into their potential. He believes it is essential to play to peoples' strengths and do whatever is necessary to help them overcome their weaknesses. The director believed that the resident had the potential to become an excellent physician; therefore, he did what he had to do to help him succeed. (See Figure 9.6 for some suggestions of ways to help people get their Solitude need met positively.)

STORY TEN

When General Pollock was a lieutenant colonel, she had an administrator on her staff who was superb in data management and analysis. She was assigned to work alone in a small, almost closet-sized office, and she was very happy in that environment. Because of her ability and some personnel losses, the operating room department director wanted to promote her into a position in the front of the office to perform the daily scheduling of the requested surgeries. These surgeries were routine and emergent in nature and required coordination with the anesthesia department, the operating room, and the surgical teams. In addition, the front area was constantly buzzing with activity, with patients coming in and out on wheeled stretchers, pharmaceutical personnel delivering requested special medication, and personnel evaluating the "board" for their assignments throughout the day. The administrator was grateful for the recognition of her abilities, but she very quickly went into distress and simply sat there unable to move to the next task without someone directing her to do it.

TEST YOUR UNDERSTANDING OF THE CONCEPTS

What is the administrator's personality type?

_____

What is her motivational need?

_____

What is her favorite channel and perception?

_____

What would you do?

_____

What would you say?

_____

What General Pollock Did

General Pollock realized the administrator was a Dreamer and needed quiet and solitude to do her work. Therefore, she addressed the environmental challenges with her and then with her supervisor. The administrator told her supervisor that she would rather have her old position, at a lower pay level, and do it well, than feel panicked because of all the noise and commotion at the front desk. The administrator thought that she could manage all the routine work if she could do it from her old office. Her supervisor agreed and it was arranged. One of the younger staff, a Promoter, was looking for more responsibility, so he asked if he could perform the coordination for the emergency procedures. This too was arranged, and the Promoter's energy ran high during those periods because he got his Incident needs met. It turned out to be an excellent solution. The Dreamer and Promoter got their needs met, both performed their new responsibilities very well, and the hospital benefited because everything ran smoothly. In addition, the timeliness of patient care improved.

STORY ELEVEN

General Pollock also told the authors about the time when, shortly after she arrived as the chief nurse anesthetist in a large medical center, a junior anesthetist timidly knocked on her open office door. When General Pollock looked up from her desk, the junior anesthetist fearfully said, "I know I am not allowed to talk with you about my leave . . ." and then burst into tears. General Pollock was stunned. She asked the anesthetist to come into the office and sit down. She asked why the anesthetist felt she could not talk with her about vacation leave requests. The anesthetist explained that in the past, staff members were not informed about leave requests until the night before it was to begin, and they were screamed at if they did ask. General Pollock asked whose policy that was, and the nurse explained that it was General Pollock's predecessor. The anesthetist explained that a close friend had asked her to be the maid of honor at her wedding and she wanted to accept. However, as a junior officer, she had to make travel arrangements early or she would not be able to afford to go to the wedding. She started crying again.

TEST YOUR UNDERSTANDING OF THE CONCEPTS

What is the junior anesthetist's personality type?

What is her motivational need?

What is her favorite channel and perception?

What would you do?

What would you say?

What General Pollock Did

General Pollock assessed the junior anesthetist as a Reactor and told her that there was a new sheriff in town. She added that she would change the old policy immediately. She also spent several minutes talking with her about what a great compliment it was to be asked to be the maid of honor. She told the anesthetist that she must be a wonderful friend and added that she had seen how caring she was in her work with her patients as well. General Pollock also told her that maintaining that caring and compassionate attitude would result in her having many friends in the hospital and that her patients would also cherish her, just as she did.

General Pollock then signed the leave paperwork so that the anesthetist could begin her travel arrangements. She also asked the anesthetist to tell the other staff members that the old rules were no longer in effect. Subsequently, General Pollock sought out opportunities to watch the anesthetist with patients and each time told her that the patients seemed very calm and trusting in their interactions with her. The anesthetist continued to need this regular reinforcement, and General Pollock continued to give it to her. From General Pollock's point of view, it was a very easy thing to do and it helped an employee enjoy being at work.

STORY TWELVE

As a cost-cutting move, a hospital in Tennessee was downgraded to a healthcare clinic. Many of the employees were given lesser positions with reduced responsibility, frequently at a reduced salary. One employee at the clinic who had been in a fairly responsible position was moved to a very small office where he had no supervisory responsibility, very little contact with other staff members, and only occasional contact with patients. In addition, his salary was reduced. He had been a useful employee, but now he was uncooperative and lethargic. He became grossly overweight, dressed very sloppily, and slept all day in his office. When he did interact with patients, he often was rude to them and was not willing to extend himself to assist them. He also was rude to fellow staff members and frequently made inappropriate sexual comments to them. In addition, he told jokes and stories that were offensive to everyone. Occasionally he attempted to get his fellow workers angry at one another by telling them that their colleagues were making negative statements about them. As a result, patients and employees frequently complained about his attitude and behavior. He was reprimanded several times and was in danger of being fired.

Because he previously had been a valuable employee and because the facility had invested a fair amount of money to provide training for him, the administrative officer at the clinic wanted to give him one last chance before terminating his employment. The administrative officer realized the employee was not getting his needs met and tried to figure out a way to help him so that he would be happy in his work, stop his negative behaviors, and improve his performance.

TEST YOUR UNDERSTANDING OF THE CONCEPTS

What is the employee's personality type?

_____

What is his motivational need?

_____

What is his favorite channel and perception?

_____

What would you do?

_____

What would you say?

_____

What the Administrative Officer Did

The administrative officer realized that the employee was a Promoter and needed action and excitement. Therefore, he decided to move him from his secluded office to a prominent location where he would be able to interact with people every day. Fortunately, the clinic had just finished a construction project and needed someone to sit at the front desk and greet people as they entered the facility, listen as they explained their medical condition, and steer them to the appropriate department. Clearly it was a risk assigning the employee to this position. However, it was a risk the administrative officer was willing to take to help salvage the employee.

The administrative officer told the employee that he personally had picked him for this position because he knew he was resourceful and persuasive and had a great deal of personal charm. He explained that these were important attributes for the person who filled the position because he would be the first face of the facility. The way he dealt with each person who came to the facility would greatly influence their impression of the facility, would shape their first opinion of the quality of service they likely would receive, and might influence their attitude toward the doctors and nurses in the facility. The administrative officer added that this was a challenge and he had selected the employee because he believed he was the best person on the staff to perform these duties.

The Result

The employee thanked the administrative officer and told him that perhaps he should get some dental work done so that his teeth would look better. He was pleased with the challenge and said he would do his best to live up to the administrative officer's confidence in him. He started once again to care about his appearance. He came to work in a dress suit, white shirt, and tie and began to greet everyone with a smile. He spoke politely to everyone, and he began to speak in a friendly way to people he had refused to speak to in several months. Staff members noted the change and reciprocated his friendliness in their interactions with him. Patients were pleased to be greeted in so friendly a manner and praised the employee for being so helpful. The employee once again was a positive influence on the staff and the patients.

The rest of the book will help healthcare providers apply the concepts in leading improvement—first in helping persuade patients to diet and lead healthier lifestyles (Chapter 10), then in leading improvement in organizations (Chapter 11).

10

Getting Patients to Diet and Lead Healthy Lifestyles

Thus far, we have focused on using the concepts of Process Communication to improve patient safety and satisfaction, and staff competence and retention. This obviously is very important. However, the big push in medicine today is to get people to be proactive in preventing illness by making healthy food choices, exercising daily, and leading healthy lifestyles. This not only improves the patient's health and energy level but also reduces healthcare costs by reducing the frequency of visits to doctors' offices and emergency rooms, and the frequency and length of hospital stays. Can the concepts of Process Communication help persuade people to become proactive in taking care of themselves? Absolutely. This chapter will explain how to do that.

Many doctors have told the authors that they know they can improve the health and longevity of their patients if they can just get them to lose weight, exercise every day, and eat healthy foods. The doctors also told the authors that they are frustrated because they feel they have failed to convince many of their patients to change their eating habits, that is, eat healthy foods and modify their lifestyles. Let's look at how a retina specialist got one of the authors, Joe, to change his lifestyle, exercise, and lose weight. Then we will explore how healthcare professionals can use these concepts to invite all their patients to modify their lifestyles.

Joe was 85 pounds overweight and was being treated for type 2 diabetes. During his annual eye examination, he was diagnosed with diabetic macular edema in his left eye and was referred to Dr. Robert Stephens, a retina specialist. Dr. Stephens ran several tests and delivered the bad news about the macular edema. He told Joe that he needed to lose one to two pounds a week, do at least a half hour of aerobic exercise every day, and lift weights a half hour each day. When Joe replied that his busy schedule did not allow him time to do all that, Dr. Stephens informed him that he had a choice. He could either follow Dr. Stephens's suggestions or face the probability of coming to see him in the future "in a wheelchair because his feet had been amputated, on dialysis because his kidneys had failed, and losing his vision." He added, "The choice is yours" and left the room to examine another patient.

Most doctors display their diplomas and citations on their office walls. The wall next to the patient's chair was empty except for one framed work, a quote from Ben Franklin: "Those who won't be counseled can't be helped." About 15 minutes later, Dr. Stephens returned to complete his examination. He asked if Joe had made a decision. Joe told him he had and would begin losing the weight and exercising immediately.

Dr. Stephens explained that the key to staying healthy is simple—build bone mass, build muscle tone, and lose body fat. He noted that weight is not the problem; excess body fat is. He explained that when people have excess body fat, they get sick. They have heart attacks and high blood pressure, and they develop diabetes. He added that physicians are starting to see teenagers with type 2 diabetes. As a result, this is the first generation since the American Revolution in which the children will not live longer than their parents. He lamented that it need not be that way. All people need to do is lose body fat, build bone mass, and build muscles. Unfortunately they don't do it.

The following week as Joe was waiting to board a plane on a business trip, he noticed a middle-aged man in a wheelchair who also was waiting to board the plane. Joe saw that both of the man's feet had been amputated and asked the man if he had been in an accident. When he replied that he had diabetes and that both feet had been amputated, Joe mentally recommitted to losing the weight and exercising. Over the next 18 months, Joe lost 65 pounds, halting his diabetic eye disease. His most recent physical examination showed no evidence of diabetes. Joe has continued to exercise and to lose weight and has now lost 75 pounds. The diabetic macular edema is still under control, and Joe's blood sugar is in the normal range, with no further indication of diabetes. According to Dr. Stephens, Joe had cured himself.

Let's look at this example from a Process Communication point of view to see why this strategy worked with Joe but might not work with another patient. Joe is a base Persister who staged through Workaholic and is in a Rebel phase. His current foreground need is Playful Contact. However, because he is a base Persister who has staged through Workaholic, he is comfortable receiving information, forming an opinion, and acting on it. As we saw in Chapter 6, Persisters are motivated by Recognition for their Work and for their Convictions. They work hard for causes they believe in and are able to stick to a task until they reach their goal. This is why this strategy was successful with Joe. The information was given to him in the Requestive channel. He heard it and formed an opinion that he needed to change his lifestyle. Once he set a goal of losing 65 pounds, he stuck to his regimen until he achieved his goal.

Unfortunately, dieting is no fun for a Rebel. Shortly after Joe achieved his goal, he reverted to his old lifestyle and began to gain weight. However, because he did not want to face the consequences Dr. Stephens had warned him about, he went back on his diet, resumed exercising, and got back to his goal weight. To maintain his weight, Joe has to find a way to get his Rebel phase need for Playful Contact met every day. That is the key. He continues to make certain he gets that need met daily so that he will continue to lead a healthy lifestyle.

Let's look at ways doctors and other healthcare professionals can apply the concepts with the other personality types. Three factors must be considered: the base and phase personality type of the patient, the way the information is communicated to the patient, and the motivation strategy. As noted in earlier chapters, people communicate best in the channel and perception preferred by their base personality type. However, they are motivated according to the needs of their phase. In Joe's case, he needed to get his need for Playful Contact met in order to stay on his diet and meet his goal. At the same time, his favorite channel is that of his Persister base personality, that is, the Requestive channel, the same channel Dr. Stephens used to communicate the information to him. He did not use the Emotive channel.

Joe usually gives his doctors copies of earlier books he and Judy have written. He gave Dr. Stephens a copy of *Communication: The Key to Effective Leadership* (ASQ Quality Press, 2009). Dr. Stephens read it and at a subsequent appointment complimented Joe on the book and asked what Joe's personality was. Joe told him, and ever since then Dr. Stephens has joked with him at the start of every appointment and uses both the Requestive and Emotive channels to communicate with him. Because he is communicating with Joe in his favorite channels and helps Joe get his need for Playful Contact met, Joe thinks he is terrific and would not consider changing doctors.

As can be seen from this example, base, phase, and any personality stages a person has gone through may have a bearing on the approach that healthcare professionals take in motivating patients to lead healthy lifestyles. For example, the strategy for a Rebel in a Rebel phase might be very different from the strategy used to motivate a Persister in a Rebel phase. Certainly, the way the information is communicated will be very different. With a Rebel in a Rebel phase, healthcare professionals should use the Emotive channel to communicate the information and should talk about likes and dislikes. At the same time, they must help the patient develop ways to get his or her Playful Contact need met. Because dieting is not fun, it may not be easy to do this. Nevertheless, if Rebel patients are not getting their contact need met in some way, they almost definitely will not stay on a diet or maintain a healthy lifestyle.

The authors have a Rebel daughter who is overweight and has just been diagnosed with type 2 diabetes. She lives in a town house with two friends. She has serious orthopedic problems and it is painful for her to exercise. Therefore, she hates exercise and does not do it. At the same time, she loves to eat candy and other unhealthy foods, and she eats more than she should at every meal. Because it is imperative that doctors find a way to reach her, the authors asked her what doctors could say to her to get her to eat healthy foods, diet, and exercise. She thought for a while and then replied, "That's a tough one. Dieting is no fun. If I could go dancing every night, I would get exercise. I might watch what I eat, then." That's the key. Dancing is fun. Regular exercise is not. As noted, the Rebel's need is to have fun. Therefore, if healthcare professionals help Rebel patients identify fun things they like doing and encourage them to do them, they have a much better chance of getting them to exercise and perhaps limit their food intake. If they can get their Rebel patients to reward themselves with a fun activity when they meet a certain weight loss—for example, one pound a week—they might be successful in getting the Rebels to stick to a weight loss program. It will not be easy, but it is the only way Rebels will change their lifestyle, short of experiencing a phase change.

In an effort to help their daughter stick to a diet, the authors made a deal with her. If she stopped eating candy, ice cream, and other sweets and lost six pounds in six weeks, they would do something special. Six weeks is a long time for a Rebel to stick to a commitment. Therefore, they set intermediate goals with appropriate rewards along the way. Because their daughter likes movies, musicals, and plays, they told her that if she lost two pounds in the first two weeks, they would take her to see a movie. If she lost another two pounds in the following two weeks, they would take her to see a play. At the end of the sixth week, they gave her a list of things to choose from as the reward for losing the weight. She met every goal, and they went to see a musical.

A *Washington Post* article described a world-class skier who, as a young girl, loved to ski fast but hated to run a mile to train.[22] According to her mother, it was torture trying to get her to run. Also, she hated to be told what to do. She insisted on doing things her way, and, as a result, some days she did very well and some days she did not. When she was older, she married a world-class skier who was a skiing technician. He tried to explain why she was inconsistent in her skiing. He said convincing her to modify her technique was difficult at first because she had already won several skiing titles and did not see the need to change her style. Also, she did not like him or anyone else telling her what to do. Eventually she listened to him and changed her technique, becoming the most successful American woman skier in history.

In the *Post* article, she is quoted as saying that sometimes she becomes a nervous wreck while waiting in line for her turn to ski in competitions. When that happens, she calls her husband and tells him she needs him. She said that he gets her to relax and calms her down by joking with her and getting her to laugh. Once she relaxes she is able to focus on her skiing and on the course. In other words, he helps her get her need for Playful Contact met and talks to her in her favorite channel, the Emotive channel. The article also quoted her mother as saying that her daughter's attitude toward training has changed completely and she now trains at a pace that amazes her teammates and competitors alike. Has she experienced a phase change? We can't say for certain, but it appears that she may have. If so, this has given her the ability to add focus to her natural talent.

There is a lesson in these stories for healthcare professionals who want to motivate patients to lose weight. Talk to them in their preferred channel of communication and find ways to help them get their needs met as a means to the end of losing weight and exercising.

Reactors are compassionate, sensitive, and warm. They perceive the world through their emotions, and they care about people. Their needs are Recognition of Person and Sensory. How can healthcare professionals use these characteristics to influence Reactor patients to lose weight and exercise? They can compliment them on their clothes, their jewelry, their hair, or some personal trait, for example, their love of and concern for their family members. Also, they can show they care about them by spending a few minutes listening when patients talk about their symptoms or their family situation. They also can encourage their patients to feel good about themselves, care about themselves, reward themselves daily, and use positive affirmations on themselves—for example, tell themselves that they are nice people and that people like them just the way they are.

In addition, Reactors need to be around people with whom they feel comfortable. Therefore, healthcare professionals can encourage them to join a support group. Because people tend to feel most comfortable with people who are like them, either at base or phase, Reactors most likely will feel comfortable in a group with many members who either are a Reactor base or are in a Reactor phase. Healthcare professionals can inform them of this and encourage them to visit several support groups in order to find a group in which they feel comfortable. Because many nurses and some doctors are Reactors, some staff members may already know of support groups made up of mainly Reactors, and they can provide this information to their Reactor patients.

Let's look at a hypothetical dialogue between a doctor and a Reactor patient who is overweight and prediabetic. First, the doctor should soften the tone of her or his voice, communicate using the Nurturative channel, and speak the language of Emotions. Presumably the doctor or a medical assistant in the office already has debriefed the patient about her or his symptoms, personal life, and lifestyle; therefore, the doctor probably understands a little about the stressors in the patient's life. Reactors need to feel that their doctor understands them and genuinely cares about them, and they must feel comfortable with their doctor and with the staff in the medical office. If they are not comfortable, they will not have confidence in the doctor and most likely will change doctors until they find someone with whom they feel they have a personal relationship. Therefore, it is important that doctors spend time with their Reactor patients in order to establish that relationship and understand enough about the patient's life and the stressors in it to be able to help their patients develop strategies to get their needs met daily.

This is not an easy thing to do, because of the insurance restrictions and the need to see a large number of patients every day. Fortunately, there is a shortcut. Dr. Kahler has developed a Key to Me Profile that doctors can use to identify the patient's personality structure, motivational needs, preferred channel of communication, and so on. The profile also explains what the person will do in distress and provides an action plan to help him or her get his or her needs met positively. The patient will feel that the doctor understands her or him, will feel comfortable with the doctor, will trust the doctor's advice, and will be more likely to maintain a healthy lifestyle. This is win–win for everyone.

Healthcare professionals should share with their patients the warning signs that they are starting to get into distress, that is, what they are likely to do in the doorway of distress. They should tell them that when they experience these warning signs, they might go off their diet unless they do something to get their needs met positively. Healthcare professionals also can tell their patients what they will do in the basement of distress and tell them that, when they find themselves doing those things, they should remind themselves that they are still good people and must engage in positive activities to get their needs met. In consulting with the patient, they also can give the patient a list of possible things she or he can do to get her or his needs met both personally and professionally.

When the patients get into distress and actually do these things, they will be amazed that their healthcare providers were able to predict their distress behaviors and provide them with possible antidotes. They will appreciate this input, will know that their healthcare provider cares about them, will be more likely to follow their provider's counsel, and will be more inclined to stay on their diet. Healthcare providers win in many ways when they do this. Their patients will be healthier; their reputation and stature will soar in the eyes of their patients; and their patients will praise their providers to their friends, relatives, and coworkers. In addition, healthcare providers will get personal satisfaction from having their patients live happier and healthier lives. The action plan in the Key to Me Profile also includes several suggestions of possible activities patients can do to get their needs met personally and professionally. Patients can tailor these suggestions to their own interests.

Patients probably will go off their diets from time to time. Healthcare professionals can warn them of this in advance and tell them that this is OK. They also should tell their patients that when this happens, they must remind themselves that they are still good people, they must do things to get their needs met, and they must go back on their diets. If they do this, their patients will be more likely to resume dieting, to exercise, and to maintain healthier lifestyles.

As we saw in Chapters 2 and 5, Promoters are very direct and prefer to communicate in the Directive channel. Therefore, doctors can be very direct with them. Promoters are also action oriented and make things happen. They are not detail people and do not want a lot of conversation. They tend to give information very concisely and prefer to receive it the same way. For this reason, healthcare professionals can give them information in bullet form without a lot of extraneous detail.

Promoters need action and excitement. They do exciting things from which they get a rush. They also make deals, and they need to look good to their peers and to those around them. Healthcare professionals can use these characteristics to their advantage in getting Promoters to change their lifestyles. For starters, Promoters will want a plan that they can start immediately and that will show quick results. Because Promoters do not stay focused on any one thing or for long periods of time, healthcare professionals can encourage Promoter patients to set short-term goals for themselves with quick rewards as they achieve them. Once each goal is reached, however, Promoter patients must set new short-term goals.

Doctors can challenge Promoter patients and encourage them to challenge themselves. Promoter patients also can make deals with themselves. To succeed in changing their lifestyles, the program they are on must be exciting and challenging. Healthcare professionals can help them achieve this goal by allowing opportunities for competition and some risk. This can be effective even if the patients compete only with themselves, for example, "I lost only one pound last week, but this week I lost two pounds."

Promoters need to be with groups of people, but they tend not to form close ties with others. Therefore, doctors can encourage attendance at support groups with drop-in programs and groups that allow intermittent attendance. This will provide Promoters an opportunity for competition and also allow them to look good to their peers. Promoters tend to do things on the spur of the moment and do not like to feel boxed in. The fact that attendance is not compulsory will be very attractive to them and will allow them to attend at the last minute, especially when they can boast of their accomplishments and make themselves look good.

What are the warning signs that Promoter patients are not getting their needs met and are in danger of going off their diets and stopping their exercise regimens? As we saw in Chapter 8, Promoters in the doorway of distress become impatient and are overly clever with others. In the basement of distress they manipulate, con, make fools of others, and try to get away with things that they know they should not do. Doctors can alert them to these behaviors and tell them that these are good warning signs that they are beginning to get into distress and need to do something to get their needs met positively. As with the other types, doctors can give their Promoter patients suggestions of activities they can do to get their needs met positively, both personally and professionally.

Dreamers are reflective, imaginative, and calm and tend not to do something until someone tells them to do it. They prefer to be alone, and they feel suffocated in the presence of a lot of people. They cannot think in a noisy environment, and they can do only one or two things at a time. Healthcare professionals can use the Directive channel with them, providing a menu for each day of the week and telling them to follow it. The menu must be specific and offer only one choice, or at most two choices, of entrée at each meal. If the menu has too many choices, Dreamer patients may not be able to choose from among the many selections. Many Dreamers do not like to exercise. But when they do, they may prefer exercises they can do alone, for example, walking, rock climbing, weight lifting, hiking, and bike riding. Doing these activities by themselves enables them to get their Solitude need met and provides them an opportunity to reflect on a wide variety of subjects.

Because Dreamers prefer to be alone, they do not need to join a support group to lose weight. Healthcare professionals can tell them the warning signs that they are starting to get into distress and can provide them with a suggested list of activities they can do to get their needs met positively. In the doorway of distress, Dreamers may start many projects but not finish any of them. Doctors can tell them that this is not a big deal, but rather a sign that they are beginning to get into distress and they must do something to get their Solitude need met. In the basement of distress, Dreamers shut down. They may just sit there and not do anything until someone tells them to do something. Again, doctors can warn Dreamers that when they see themselves doing any of these behaviors, it is a warning sign that they must get their needs met or they probably will not stay on their diets and probably will not exercise.

As we saw in earlier chapters, Persisters need to be respected and prefer to communicate in the Requestive channel. Healthcare professionals can establish rapport with them by giving them information, telling them they admire their commitment to their weight loss and exercise program, and asking their opinion of things they believe in. They also have a need for Recognition for Work; therefore, medical personnel can compliment them on their weight loss, their improved muscle tone, and the improvement in their medical test results. They also can encourage Persisters to think for themselves, plan a strategy, record and chart their progress, and understand dietary and health information. Persisters respond best to exchanges of facts, information, and opinions. Therefore, medical personnel can ask questions that invite thinking and opinions. This includes inviting Persister patients to participate in all aspects of planning and goal setting. Because Persisters prefer one-on-one relationships, doctors and nurses can encourage them to use a buddy system for support. These simple steps will go a long way to enabling Persisters to maintain their changing lifestyles.

As we saw in Chapter 8, when Persisters enter the doorway of distress they become critical of others and focus on what others are doing wrong. They may also focus on what they themselves are doing wrong; for example, they may get very critical of themselves if they go off their diet or stop exercising.

Healthcare professionals can invite them out of their doorway of distress by asking their opinion of things, for example, asking them why they believe they stopped dieting and what they think it would take to get them to resume their diet. They also can tell them that this is not a big deal, as long as they renew their commitment and resume their dietary regimen.

In the basement of distress, Persisters attack others and push their beliefs onto those who do not agree with them. Frequently this will be with people they love or to whom they are close. This will compound their distress and may result in their going into the cellar of distress. In the cellar of distress, Persister patients may give up on others, for example, their healthcare providers, because they feel they can't trust them. They also may give up on their diet or exercise program because they believe there is no use in continuing. When this happens, they may criticize their healthcare providers because they may come to lose respect for them. Healthcare professionals can invite them out of their basements or cellars by helping them get their Conviction and Recognition for Work needs met positively. They may be able to head off this criticism by telling their Persister patients the warning signs that they are starting to get into distress and explaining to them what they will do in second-degree distress. When their Persister patients actually do these things, they will have much more respect for their caregivers, which will prompt them to resume dieting and to lead a healthier lifestyle.

As we saw in the example of the authors' daughter, dieting is not fun. However, because Rebels are motivated by fun activities, it is crucial that they find a way to make it fun if they are going to change their lifestyle. If they can't find a way to make dieting fun, Rebels likely will not stick to a diet for any great length of time. In the doorway of distress, Rebels may experience dieting as being difficult, will struggle over small matters more than they need to, and will experience a period of indecisiveness. They may feel cornered and may begin to feel that they have no good options. For example, they may feel they are damned if they don't stay on their diet, because they will get sick; but at the same time, they are damned if they do stick to their diet, because they won't have any fun. They also may expect others to help them stick to their diet. If this does not happen, they may go into their basement of distress and begin to blame others for their inability to stay on their diet or to exercise. Healthcare professionals can tell them that these typical reactions are warning signs that they need to find ways to get their need for Playful Contact met or they will not be able to stick to their diet.

In the basement of distress, Rebel patients may refuse to take responsibility for not staying on their diet, may complain and find fault with their diet or exercise program, may focus on reasons why their diet or exercise program won't work, and may start arguments with their healthcare providers just for the sake of disagreeing with them. When this happens, healthcare providers can suggest fun ways their Rebel patients can get their Playful Contact need met. One way they can do this is to communicate with their Rebel patients in the Emotive channel. Just hearing the upbeat tone of this channel often is enough to get Rebels out of distress.

It is almost impossible for healthcare workers to give Workaholic patients too much information, as they want to know as much as possible about their condition and possible courses of action. Moreover, they want the information delivered in a logical sequence in the Requestive channel. Their needs are Recognition for Work and Time Structure. The latter need is so acute that the authors have seen Workaholic patients leave doctors' offices when they have been kept waiting beyond what they consider to be a reasonable length of time. Because of their need for Recognition for Work, Workaholics need to be congratulated for the weight they have lost, their determination to live a healthier life, and their efforts to stay on their diet and to exercise. Healthcare professionals can give them facts and help them see the logical consequences if they do not lose weight, eat healthy foods, and exercise. They can ask their Workaholic patients questions about their lifestyle and have them give reasons why they should change their lifestyle. Doctors and nurses can be very blunt in describing the consequences if the Workaholic patients do not go on a diet and do not start exercising. They also can ask their Workaholic patients questions and get suggestions of ways they can implement a healthier lifestyle.

In the doorway of distress, Workaholic patients may make complicated statements and use big words in convoluted sentences when describing their condition to their healthcare provider. They also may put off doing things for pleasure because they have to stick to their diet, or they may put off exercising because they have so much work to do that they do not have time to exercise. If they are often putting off doing things for personal pleasure, they may get into distress about being on a diet. Healthcare providers can tell their Workaholic patients that if they find themselves doing this, they must do something to get their needs met. The providers also can help their Workaholic patients come up with several ideas of ways they can get their needs met.

If they do not get themselves out of distress at this point, they may go into the basement of distress. Here, Workaholic patients may start orally attacking others, especially those close to them, because they don't know how to think, are not organized, or are not on time. This could include their care providers and members of the providers' office staffs. When this happens, healthcare providers can invite their patients out of distress by giving them a battery charge for the motivational need that corresponds to the behavior their patients are showing.

Patients of all six types who are not getting their phase needs met probably will not continue to maintain a healthy lifestyle. Therefore, healthcare professionals must ensure that the motivation strategy is geared to help their patients get their phase needs met positively. Preferably, the strategy also will enable patients to get their base needs met. In any case, healthcare professionals should communicate with their patients in the same channel that corresponds to that preferred by their base personality type (see Chapter 5). With base Rebels, it is the Emotive channel; with base Reactors, the Nurturative channel; with base Workaholics and Persisters, the Requestive channel; and with base Dreamers and Promoters, the Directive channel.

The importance of helping patients develop strategies to get their base and phase motivational needs met as the key to helping them maintain a healthy lifestyle cannot be stressed enough. When patients get their needs met positively, they are more likely to have a positive attitude toward life and will be more able to deal positively with the stressors in their lives. This, in turn, will result in their being more open to accepting change and will make it easier for healthcare administrators and healthcare leaders to implement quality improvement measures, thereby improving patient safety and satisfaction.

11

Using the Concepts in Leading Improvement

People in many sectors of society insist that the health-care system must be changed, the quality of patient care and patient safety must be improved, medical expenses must be reduced, and more people must be insured. Consequently, these are tumultuous times for healthcare professionals. Indeed, many of these and other changes are under way. However, change is uncomfortable for many people. Therefore, people frequently resist change and get into distress when changes are made. When people talk about change, what they really want is improvement. If the need for improvement is communicated clearly to people and if, at the same time, they are shown how they will benefit from the improvements, it is easier to involve people in bringing these improvements about. This is especially true when introducing a quality program at a healthcare facility or system. This chapter will discuss how this has been done in various medical facilities using the concepts of Dr. Kahler's Process Communication Model.®

LEADING IMPROVEMENT IN A NATIONAL HEALTHCARE SYSTEM

Ascension Health is the largest nonprofit healthcare system in the United States, with 107,000 employees in 69 hospitals and several assisted-living facilities in 20 states and the District of Columbia. Ascension was committed to reducing the number of accidents, including accidental deaths, throughout its healthcare system. Two of the biggest hurdles it faced in accomplishing this were the many different healthcare culture groups and the huge communication gaps between them.

To explore the extent of the differences in the various cultural groups, questionnaires were sent out on three occasions, and 30,000 were returned each time. The questionnaires showed that doctors were twice as optimistic as nurses, and administrators were twice as optimistic as doctors. Ninety percent of the doctors who use the hospitals are not employees of the hospital. They are private-practice physicians, and they make most of the healthcare decisions for their patients. Time is an issue for them. They have patients to see, and they do not want to spend time in meetings at the hospital. As a result, miscommunication is a common problem among the hospital administrators, the doctors who use the hospital, and other caregivers. Miscommunication also was occurring between some of the doctors and some of the nurses due to the differences in their personality types. Clearly, there was a need to improve communication throughout the healthcare system.

To bridge these gaps, the organization did many things. In 2003, it set goals of greatly reducing the number of preventable accidents and of eliminating accidental deaths in five years. Dr. David Pryor, the chief medical officer of the system, chose the Process Communication Model® as a vehicle to improve communication through the clinical leadership of the healthcare system and had his staff, the clinical excellence team (who provided clinical leadership for the system), and his departments trained in the concepts. The system also standardized its processes by adopting many of the recommendations contained in two books published by the Institute of Medicine, *To Err Is Human* (1999) and *Crossing the Quality Chasm*

(2001), and by using bundles of standard practices based on proven efficacy.

Dr. Pryor found that the concepts of Process Communication facilitated communication of the goals so that everyone understood them. Particularly in communicating with caregivers, it is important to use the correct channel. Using the correct channel and perception is also important in improving communication with patients. When working with caregivers, he found that the Requestive channel was effective but the Directive channel was not. There are times, however, when caregivers use the Directive channel, for example, in resuscitating patients. After his staff members were trained in the Process Communication concepts, their communication skills improved in their dealings with one another, with their staff members, and with healthcare providers. Their teamwork also improved because, as they better understood how their colleagues viewed the world and the basis for their positions and recommendations, they were more patient in their dealings with one another and with everyone with whom they interacted.

Dr. Pryor also individualized the way he motivated his staff members and patients by helping them get their motivational needs met positively. This was useful in influencing them not only to accept change but also to want to implement it. Whenever he talked to a group, he made certain that he helped everyone in the group get his or her needs met. He complimented everyone for the improvements and individualized the way he said it so that everyone got his or her needs met. For example, he noted the improvement and then praised people for their hard work (for the Workaholics and Persisters), their commitment and dedication (for the Persisters), and their concern for their patients and for one another (for the Reactors). Because Dreamers need solitude and time to reflect on issues, he always gave them an opportunity to get their Solitude need met and time to reflect on possible courses of action before asking for their input. He did this in several ways. He might give them advance notice of topics to be discussed on which he wanted their input, or he might present the issue at a meeting and then give them time to think about it and provide input at a subsequent meeting. He also gave patients battery charges for their psychological needs whenever he dealt with them.

Dr. Pryor also helped people get their motivational needs met positively whenever he mentored them. For example, one day a very senior person, a Persister, was in a meeting with a team of people who were going to implement a program to input data electronically. He knew more about the program than anyone in the room and he laid out all the problems in an Autocratic interaction style. The meeting disintegrated. Afterward, Dr. Pryor gave the senior staff member a battery charge for his Conviction need by telling him, "You are right." He then used the Requestive channel to allow the senior staff member to understand why things disintegrated. He asked him, "Were you effective? Did anything change as a result of your interaction?" By first giving the battery charge, Dr. Pryor knew that the senior person would be more likely to accept the message that he needed to use a more Democratic interaction style if he wanted to be effective. By using the Requestive channel to counsel him, he knew the senior staff member was more likely to understand the need to change. The senior staff member heard the message and improved his communication and relationships with the team members.

LEADING INNOVATION IN A HEALTHCARE SYSTEM MEDICAL EDUCATION DEPARTMENT

A Reactor nurse educator at a Tennessee hospital was in charge of medical education for the doctors, nurses, and staff members. She also was accountable for all the activity planners performing their planning according to the regulations and guidelines. Because she is a Reactor and wanted everyone to like her, she found it very difficult to hold her peers accountable. Consequently, she was in second- and third-degree distress every day for several months. She spent a lot of time alone and avoided interacting with her coworkers because she hated having to confront them and wanted to avoid conflict. In addition, she made mistakes and created a lot of stress in the hospital. She was also under a lot of pressure from her supervisor and she began to hate her job.

After she learned the concepts of Process Communication she understood that she was in severe distress. She was able to see what she was doing to sabotage herself and how she was setting herself up for failure. More important, she understood that she had to find ways to get her motivational needs met so that she could be productive. She used the concepts to get herself out of distress and turn things around. She started by making an effort to connect with her coworkers and rebuild her relationships with them. Once she accepted the fact that confrontation was difficult for her because of her personality type and that it was OK to feel that way, she realized she was still a valuable employee who had other strengths and many other things that she did very well. She began to think clearly and was able to help all the people around her get their needs met positively.

Her relations with her supervisor and her colleagues improved dramatically. So did the performance of her duties. When she spoke with her coworkers about things that had to be done, they performed better because of the improved relationships, because she was the person helping them get their needs met, and because she individualized the way she communicated with them. They were able to understand what she was saying even when she was telling them things they did not want to hear. This translated into improved processes in the hospital.

A short time later, new standards and guidelines were established for medical education, and the hospital was not compliant with them. The hospital was up for reaccreditation, and major changes in the medical education program at the hospital had to be made in a very short time. The nurse educator was responsible for effecting the change. It was important that the hospital get reaccredited to provide continuing medical education. If the hospital did not get reaccredited, it might not have been able to provide medical education. This would have been a serious problem because, if the doctors and nurses could not get their continuing education credits there, they would have to go elsewhere for their training. In that case, the doctors might stop using the hospital to treat their patients, resulting in a considerable loss of revenue.

To meet the new standards, people had to do several new things that they were not used to doing. In addition, all the new requirements were imposed on them at once. There was additional paperwork, they had to evaluate educational activities and programs, they had to have speakers fill out financial disclosure forms, and so on. Everyone, including her supervisor, was in distress for fear of losing the accreditation. The nurse educator felt certain that she would not have been able to bring about all the necessary changes without her new communication skills and without her newly improved relations with her coworkers and her supervisor.

To prepare for the accreditation review, the nurse educator had to persuade the activity coordinators of the need to meet the new requirements and get them to actually do the extra work required. She sent out a general letter to all of them explaining what they had to do to comply with the new standards, but that did not work. Therefore, she met with each one individually. Every meeting was different because she individualized the way she communicated with them. She gave each of them a battery charge for their needs at the beginning of each meeting and repeatedly throughout. She also communicated with each person in that person's preferred channel and perception. This immediately reduced the distress level and helped her persuade all the activity coordinators to want to implement the changes.

The changes were implemented before the reaccreditation visit, and the hospital medical education program was reaccredited. The doctors, who are the customers of the hospital, were happy because they could get their continuing education credits at the hospital. The nurse educator was pleased that her efforts to bring about major improvement in the way medical education is run at the hospital were successful.

LEADING IMPROVEMENT AT A MEDICAL FACILITY

Because of the downturn in the economy, an Alabama hospital was forced to reduce the size of its staff. The board of directors also decided to reduce the number of services offered and reduce the facility from a hospital to a smaller medical facility as a cost-cutting measure. As a result of the reduction, many of the positions were downgraded, and people who were retained on staff were given new, frequently lesser responsibilities. This resulted in a serious morale problem for the administration.

Every month the facility administrator held a general staff conference. After the downsizing, the conference sessions were unruly as staff members challenged the administrator on various issues and vehemently disagreed with his position on many things. They frequently orally attacked the administrator, and the conferences usually turned into gripe sessions. As a result, people hated attending the conferences. To try to improve staff morale, the administrator suggested they have the staff trained in the concepts of Process Communication.

The training was done over a period of about 15 months. As more and more people were trained, they became more understanding of one another and more respectful of other people's positions on the issues. The atmosphere at the conferences slowly changed. According to one administrative officer at the facility, the tipping point came after about half the staff members had received Process Communication training and began applying the concepts in their dealings with one another. By the time everyone received the training, the staff members had stopped their attacks during the conferences. The atmosphere at the conferences has now completely improved. People are more respectful of one another and deal with one another collegially. Everyone is pleased with the improved atmosphere.

The administrative officer stated that he has noticed that when people start to get angry during a discussion, others will politely ask them what distress mask they are wearing. When this happens, the speaker will stop and ask for confirmation that he or she has a distress mask on. When others confirm that the speaker is wearing a mask, the speaker completely changes his or her behavior and begins communicating in a normal manner. This has gone a long way in improving the morale of the staff members and their effectiveness in dealing with their patients and with one another.

Whenever the authors return to the facility to do additional training, people who have received the training are always happy to see them, they greet them with a smile, and welcome them back to the facility. Many staff members thank them for helping them communicate more effectively with people with whom they previously had difficulty dealing. Many of the staff members come to the authors with a specific problem and ask for their advice on how to deal with a difficult situation.

Frequently, participants in the seminars ask for specific strategies they can use to help them communicate more effectively with their children and spouses. When they apply the suggested strategies at home, their relationships with the children who have been frustrating them improve dramatically. Many times they ask their spouses to help them get their psychological needs met positively. When their spouses respond and help them get their needs met, the staff members are better able to deal positively with the issues facing them at home. This reduces the pressure on them, making them happier at home and happier, healthier, and more effective at work. As a result, they are better able to focus on providing higher-quality service to their patients at the facility.

LEADING IMPROVEMENT IN A FAMILY CLINIC

Wendy Potter, who was introduced in Chapter 6, and Dr. Sue Geier are two of the four partners in the Child and Family Consulting Clinic in Melbourne, Florida. They use the concepts of Process Communication every day in managing their clinical practice and in dealing with their patients and the family members of their patients. The partners have a meeting every Tuesday at 12:30. Two of the partners are Reactors, one is a Rebel, and one is a Workaholic. They all have different perceptions of what they should be doing and how they should deal with the various issues they discuss. They talk out all of the issues with everyone staying up in their condominium—that is, dealing with one another positively. They help all of the partners get their needs met in every meeting and individualize the way they communicate with each other. As a result, they arrive at consensus on every issue. They frequently disagree during the discussions, but there is no animosity.

They also use these concepts in personnel selection and in dealing with their staff members. Prior to interviewing a candidate for a specific position, Dr. Geier and Potter decide what strengths the candidate must have to perform the expected tasks well. Having agreed on this, they decide the personality type and possibly the phase of their ideal candidate. Armed with this information, they then conduct their interviews. During the interview, they use all four channels and all six perceptions in talking with the candidate. This helps them understand the candidate's personality structure. They also listen for indications of first-degree distress to confirm their diagnosis of that structure. In this way, they usually find a good fit for the position.

Sometimes the person they hire appears to be a good fit but turns out not to be. In those instances when it is necessary to let an employee go, they also use the concepts so that there is a happy separation. For example, one employee, a Reactor in a Rebel phase, had no energy and was inefficient. She was getting no work done and expected everyone else to do her work for her. They did everything they could to help her get her psychological needs met positively, but her job performance did not improve. Finally, they decided they were going to have to terminate her employment. In talking with her, they helped her get her Recognition of Person need met positively by telling her that she was a very nice person and they liked having her in the office. They added that they felt they were asking her to do too much. When she agreed that they were giving her too much to do, they told her that this was not fair to her and, therefore, they were going to let her go. The employee thanked them and left happily with her self-esteem intact.

In dealing with patients and their family members, Dr. Geier and Potter constantly had to remind patients' parents of the clinic rules. For example, certain areas of the clinic are off-limits, but parents and some children continued to enter those spaces. How could they get them to stay out of the private spaces, such as the freezers and the medical file room? How could they keep them from putting dirty diapers in the trash cans and persuade them to put them in the diaper pails instead? They decided to individualize the way they spoke to each of the parents and to the children and give them battery charges for their psychological needs as they explained the rules and the reasons for them. Almost immediately the situation improved.

Everyone stayed out of the private spaces, and they put the dirty diapers in the diaper pails. Dr. Geier and Potter communicate this way every day with everyone who enters the clinic. As a result, the clinic runs very smoothly.

LEADING IMPROVEMENT IN A HEALTHCARE SYSTEM EDUCATION INSTITUTE

Barbette Weimer-Elder is executive director of the Education Institute in Adventist Healthcare, part of a global healthcare system for the Seventh Day Adventist Church.

In 2005, the employee engagement baseline for her team was very low. She had read a report on publicly traded companies published by the Gallup Organization that indicated those organizations with top-quartile employee engagement had 2.6 times higher earnings-per-share growth than companies with below-average engagement. Therefore, she decided to set a goal of bringing her team to high employee engagement as a strategy to increase business outcomes. The Gallup report also stated that those business units with top-quartile rankings had 12% higher customer loyalty, 18% higher productivity, and 12% higher profitability. In contrast, bottom-quartile business units, when compared with top-quartile units, had 31%–51% higher turnover, 51% more "inventory shrinkage," and 62% more accidents. This reinforced her commitment to improve employee engagement in her team.

Weimer-Elder was aware that there was a lack of clear communication within her team. Therefore, she decided to attend a Process Communication seminar to see if she could use the concepts to improve employee engagement in her team. After attending the seminar and returning to her office, she began individualizing the way she communicated with each of her team members using their preferred channel and perception. She was pleasantly surprised at the immediate improvement in her communication with her team members. She also helped them get their needs met positively every day, and when they got into distress, she used the concepts successfully to invite them out of unproductive behavior so that they once again engaged positively and were productive. As a result, she was successful in moving the team through serious conflict resolution stages. From then on, disagreements were expressed in positive ways within the department, and the conflict resolution process was viewed positively and valued. All members of the team felt comfortable stating their positions very positively, and each team member was trusted as a key contributor to the productivity of the team.

As she became more proficient in applying the concepts, Weimer-Elder began to use an individualistic leadership style, in which she used the Autocratic, Democratic, Benevolent, and Laissez Faire styles with the people who responded best to each of them. As she shifted her styles, she began to see many elements of employee engagement improve in the department. As a result of her personal success, she began having her team members learn the concepts. Communication among team members has improved, and they are more engaged and more productive. In addition, the team has scored in the top quartile of the Gallup healthcare database for four consecutive years.

LEADING CHANGE TO DEVELOP A TEAM

When an administrator took over a department at a Florida hospital, staff morale was very low, staff turnover was very high, and there was no teamwork among the staff members. In spite of this, patient satisfaction was very high. The administrator wondered how this could be and decided to watch her staff very carefully to try to understand what was happening in the department that produced such disparate results. The administrator noticed that one of her nurses (a Rebel) always was able to establish great relationships with patients and doctors. In fact, she was the only nurse to whom the doctors talked. The other nurses were present but were largely ignored by the patients and by the doctors. Also, the nurse was very dramatic and tended to act like a queen bee in the department. Moreover, she had a tendency to be very blunt in her statements to patients and to other staff members. For example, she would enter a patient's room, find out that a nurse on another shift had not given a patient her or his medication, and say something like, "I can't believe the nurse on the other shift didn't give you your meds." As a result, patients came to question the professionalism of the other staff members. The nurse also had a tendency to criticize the other staff members and complain to her supervisor that they didn't know what they were doing, had not been well trained in nursing school, and so forth. Naturally, this had a negative impact on the other staff members and it was destroying team cohesion. In fact, the department was not functioning as a team but as one member with several bit players. Because of the impact the nurse was having on the other staff members, the senior members of the nursing staff wanted to fire her.

The administrator did not want to do this, because she recognized the nurse's strengths and the positive relationships she had with the patients. She realized that if she could get the nurse to see what her attitude was doing to the other members of the staff, she might be able to use the nurse's enthusiasm and expertise to get the department functioning as a team, thereby improving staff satisfaction and patient safety. The administrator decided to attach herself to the nurse, and she began using the Emotive channel in communicating with her. She also looked for ways to help the nurse have fun during the workday so that she got her Playful Contact need met every day. After she established a relationship with the nurse so that the nurse began to like her, she started talking to the nurse about her comments and about ways to improve teamwork within the department.

When the administrator heard the nurse make a negative comment about another nurse or staff member, she spoke to her and asked her if she realized the negative impact those statements had on the other staff members. Specifically, she asked how the nurse would like it if someone made those statements about her. The nurse had not thought about the impact her statements might have and agreed to stop making them. In this way, the administrator got the nurse to change her behavior toward the other staff members. This had the ancillary benefit of opening up the lines of communication between the nurse and the administrator. With the lines of communication open, the administrator asked the nurse if she would be willing to run the training program for the department and use her experience to help train all the new nurses. The nurse agreed.

The nurse quickly established the same relationships with the new nurses as she had with the patients. The new nurses respect her years of experience and they love her freewheeling style. Because they are her protégés, she does everything she can to tutor them and help them become more proficient healthcare providers. As a result, the department now functions as a very effective team, morale and staff satisfaction are high, and patient satisfaction and patient safety are at all-time highs. The nurse is happy, the administrator is happy, the other staff members are happy, the patients are delighted, and the doctors who use the hospital are very happy. Clearly this is a win–win situation for everyone.

LEADING CHANGE IN A WOMEN'S HOSPITAL

Dr. Constance Battle, who was introduced in Chapter 3, is the former CEO of Women's Hospital in Washington, DC. The senior management team was made up of a Dreamer, a

Persister, a Rebel, a Promoter, and a Reactor. In order for the team to function well, Dr. Battle had to individualize the way she communicated with them. She tried to ensure that each of them got their needs met positively every day and was successful with all except the Promoter. Dr. Battle believed that if the team were to function cohesively, the members had to be able to trust one another. For that to happen, she believed they had to get to know one another well. Therefore, at a team meeting, she had each member of the team tell the other team members the key indicators about themselves. They also shared funny stories about themselves to help the Rebel get his need for Playful Contact met positively and because she wanted the Rebel to enjoy attending the meetings. She believed he would be happier in a lighthearted atmosphere. She also helped the Promoter get his Incident need met. Each person was valued and validated according to his or her needs, and Dr. Battle spent time one on one with each of them. In these personal meetings she individualized the way she dealt with them.

During the meetings she told them that she expected they would not agree on everything and that when they disagreed, she wanted to hear their point of view and the reasons they held a particular view. In addition, she told them that when there was disagreement during a discussion, they should not take it personally. It also did not mean that they were not valued members of the team. This strategy worked well for all members of the team except the Promoter, and all except the Promoter have continued to maintain their friendships to this day.

The number of patients at the hospital was increasing dramatically, so the team decided they had to enlarge the hospital and increase the size of the hospital staff by 40%. So that the board would have confidence in the team, Dr. Battle introduced each of the team members to the members of the board and had each of them brief the board on their areas of responsibility. This also was an opportunity to help the

Promoter get his Incident need met by giving him a chance to look good to the board members. Unfortunately, the Promoter was in severe distress and used this introduction to improve his position with the members of the board and to sabotage the relationships the other members of the executive team had with them. As a result, the board members lost confidence in the executive team and replaced them. This illustrates the importance of ensuring that everyone gets their psychological needs met positively and the possible consequences if they do not.

It is especially important when leaders deal with the public—for example, when they try to convince the public of their position on issues or of the quality service their hospital provides—that they include in their public presentations something in each of the six perceptions and speak in all four channels. In this way, everyone will be more inclined to listen to them and will understand clearly what they are saying. They also should include battery charges for all six types in their presentations. Above all, leaders cannot allow themselves to be in distress when they address a group, and they cannot allow themselves to be provoked into putting on a distress mask when addressing a group. Indeed, they should not allow themselves to be in distress whenever they interact with another person, but this is especially true when trying to persuade people to their point of view.

As we saw in Chapter 3, people do not want to be talked down to by "arrogant, condescending" people. When many leaders get into distress, they are inviting people to perceive them as pompous and arrogant. In addition, as we saw in Chapters 5 and 8, 85% of people in North America do not like to be told what to do. Therefore, if leaders use an Autocratic interaction style, many people may feel that they are being attacked or that the leader is talking down to them. For these reasons, healthcare professionals must limit their use of the Autocratic style in their presentations.

Forgoing an Autocratic interaction style is helpful in all interpersonal relationships, but it is especially helpful in persuading people to accept change. It is also essential when attempting to facilitate improvement in the quality of service provided in healthcare facilities. Improving the quality of care in a healthcare facility cannot be imposed from above, because most people resent being told that they have to do something. They want an opportunity to express their views and be heard. This is especially true in situations requiring major change. Because improving the quality of healthcare and developing a culture of patient safety require extensive change in the culture of the facility as well as standardizing the processes, even minor changes are uncomfortable and stressful.

Changing the culture of a healthcare facility is especially stressful and frequently results in employees getting into distress. When that happens, some people aggressively resist any changes; others attempt to sabotage the changes so that they can say, "I told you it wouldn't work." Still others try to disrupt the process of change by getting team members to distrust one another. Others get confused and make mistakes, thereby reducing the quality of care, and still others shut down and don't do anything until someone tells them what to do.

A recent example of what happens when "experts" try to dictate change is the release of a study by the U.S. Preventive Services Task Force in 2009, recommending that women delay having routine mammograms for the early detection of breast cancer until after age 50. The study also recommended that women have mammograms less frequently. As a result of the uproar that followed, the American Cancer Society issued a press release on November 19, 2009, stating that it would not change its recommendation of annual mammography after age 40. If the public had been able to participate in discussions prior to the release of the report and had been educated on the findings in advance, the uproar might have been avoided.

INFLUENCING IMPROVEMENT IN SAFETY PROCEDURES IN BIOMEDICAL RESEARCH LABORATORIES

Dr. Jonathan Richmond is the former director of the Office of Health and Safety at the Centers for Disease Control and Prevention (CDC). When he was at the CDC, he was charged with improving safety in biomedical research facilities within the CDC in Atlanta and at other federal locations. As the number of biomedical research facilities increased, so did the scope of Dr. Richmond's responsibilities and the number of people assigned to his department. Their mission was to persuade very intelligent, well-educated, and highly opinionated scientists to adopt and follow rather stringent safety measures in their research laboratories. To accomplish this mission, Richmond realized that he and his staff needed to be able to communicate their message clearly to a diverse group of people in ways that would result in their seeing the need for the safety procedures and being willing to adhere to them. He learned the concepts of Process Communication and decided to use these concepts as the vehicle to fulfill his responsibilities.

Dr. Richmond began applying the concepts of Process Communication with his staff members, individualizing the way he managed, communicated with, and motivated them. To this end, he helped them get their needs met positively every day. As communication improved and as his staff members got their needs met positively, they became a more cohesive team, they were happier in their work, and their productivity increased. To improve their ability to communicate with their clients, Dr. Richmond had them all trained in the Process Communication concepts. They then used the concepts to establish relationships with their clients. They individualized the way they communicated with them, gave the people they were dealing with battery charges for their psychological needs, and spoke to them using the other person's favorite channel and perception. As a result, they were very successful in persuading their clients to adopt effective safety measures for their facilities.

Dr. Richmond is currently the CEO of Jonathan Richmond Associates. In his present position, he is a biosafety consultant to governments in Asia, Africa, and Latin America that are setting up biohazard medical research programs. He also consults with companies that are constructing biomedical laboratories. He believes it is critically important that they maintain very high safety standards in their laboratories, and he uses the concepts of Process Communication in all of his dealings with government officials, scientists, researchers, engineers, and corporate executives in these countries. He believes that unless these scientists follow stringent safety procedures, the research in these facilities could have disastrous consequences. Therefore, he considers it critically important that he succeed in his efforts to persuade them to adhere to these procedures. He has found the concepts of Process Communication very useful in achieving this goal.

Healthcare professionals can greatly improve the likelihood that their employees will embrace change if they use an individualistic interaction style in proposing it. They can give the Reactors an opportunity to express their feelings and reassure them that they are part of the organization "family." They can provide complete information for the Workaholics and give them an opportunity to provide input. Quality, standards, and value are important to Persisters. Therefore, healthcare administrators can explain how the changes being proposed will improve the quality of healthcare in the facility, will raise the standards, and will add value. They also can ask the Persisters for their opinions of the various proposals. They can use a Laissez Faire style with the Rebels and make sure they have an opportunity to tell everyone what they like and do not like about the procedures being considered. Above all, healthcare professionals can make certain that they periodically inject some humor into the meetings. Additionally, they can tell the Promoters how they will benefit personally from the change and give them an opportunity to look good. Finally, they can give the Dreamers time to think about the changes contemplated and actively solicit their ideas. If leaders do this, staff members will be much more willing to endorse the need for change and to support improving the quality of the services they provide.

Epilogue

The stories in this book demonstrate what is possible when healthcare professionals establish relationships with everyone with whom they interact. Knowing how to individualize the way they communicate with their patients will ensure that their patients hear and understand the information and instructions the healthcare professionals are giving them. In addition, when healthcare providers help patients get their motivational needs met positively, they establish positive relationships with their patients and help their patients stay out of distress. This is win–win for everyone. The patients will have a positive attitude toward their healthcare providers and will be more likely to be able to deal with their medical condition positively. This frequently will result in patients recovering faster. In all likelihood, the patients will praise their healthcare providers to their family and friends, thereby generating positive publicity for the institution and for their providers. This in turn will create more business for the healthcare providers and for the institution. Healthcare providers also will get greater satisfaction from seeing their patients recover faster. In addition, this may result in their patients deciding to lead a healthier lifestyle.

When healthcare administrators and healthcare managers use an individualistic management or interaction style in leading and managing their departments or their facilities and also individualize the way they communicate with and motivate their staff members, the staff members will be happier and more effective. This usually results in the staff members being able to deal with the daily stressors that occur in handling emergencies as they arise without getting into distress. When this happens, the staff members are more likely to be able to focus on providing quality care to their patients. This, plus using quality tools to systematize all processes, will greatly improve patient safety and patient satisfaction. This, again, is a win–win for everyone.

Finally, when healthcare providers individualize the way they communicate with and motivate their family members and friends, their relationships with their family members and friends will improve. This will relieve a great deal of distress at home and ensure that the healthcare providers are coming to work in a positive place. This, again, is a win–win for everyone. Family members will be happier, family relationships will be stronger, and the healthcare providers will be more effective in dealing with their patients and with their colleagues.

Happy processing.

Notes

1. Institute of Medicine, *To Err Is Human: Building a Safer Health System* (Washington, DC: National Academy Press, 2000).

2. HealthGrades, *HealthGrades Patient Safety in American Hospitals Study*, March 2011, http://www.healthgrades.com/business/img/HealthGradesPatientSafetyInAmericanHospitalsStudy2011.pdf.

3. Sir Liam Donaldson and Pauline Philip, "Patient Safety—a Global Priority," *Bulletin of the World Health Organization* 82, no. 12 (2004), http://www.who.int/bulletin/volumes/82/12/editorial11204html/en/.

4. Institute of Medicine, *The Safe Use Initiative and Health Literacy: A Workshop*, December 2010, http://www.iom.edu/Reports/2010/The-Safe-Use-Initiative-and-Health-Literacy-A-Workshop.aspx.

5. R. Douglas Scott II, *The Direct Medical Costs of Healthcare-Associated Infections in U.S. Hospitals and the Benefits of Prevention*, March 2009, Centers for Disease Control and Prevention, http://www.cdc.gov/ncidod/dhqp/pdf/Scott_CostPaper.pdf.

6. C. P. Landrigan, G. J. Parry, C. B. Bones, A. D. Hackbarth, D. A. Goldman, and P. J. Sharek, "Temporal Trends in Rates of Patient Harm Resulting from Medical Care," *New England Journal of Medicine* 363, no. 22 (2010): 2124–2134.

7. Robert Q. Watson and Ken Leeson, "On the Clock," ASQ *Quality Progress*, March 2011, http://asq.org/quality-progress/2011/03/best-practices/on-the-clock.html.

8. Jody Hoffer Gittell, *High Performance Healthcare: Using the Power of Relationships to Achieve Quality, Efficiency and Resilience* (New York: McGraw-Hill, 2009), 13.

9. Gittell, *High Performance Healthcare*, 30.

10. Gittell, *High Performance Healthcare*, 35.

11. Taibi Kahler, *The Mastery of Management*, 4th ed. (Little Rock, AR: Kahler Communications, 2000), 54–55.

12. Kaja Whitehouse, "Why CEOs Need to Be Honest with Their Boards," *Wall Street Journal*, January 14, 2008.

13. Margaret Race, "Evaluation of the Public Review Process and Risk Communication at High-Level Biocontainment Laboratories," *Applied Biosafety* 13, no. 1 (2008): 45.

14. R. Lofstedt, "Good and Bad Examples of Siting and Building Biosafety Level Four Laboratories: A Study of Winnipeg, Galveston, and Etobicoke," *Journal of Hazardous Materials* 93, no. 1 (2002): 47–66, quoted in Race, note 13.

15. Race, "Evaluation of the Public Review Process," 50.

16. Race, "Evaluation of the Public Review Process," 54.

17. Judith Ann Pauley and Joseph F. Pauley, *Communication: The Key to Effective Leadership* (Milwaukee, WI: ASQ Quality Press, 2009); Judith Ann Pauley, Dianne F. Bradley, and Joseph F. Pauley, *Here's How to Reach Me: Matching Instruction to Personality Types in Your Classroom* (Baltimore, MD: Brookes Publishing Company, 2002).

18. Tom V. Savage, *Discipline for Self-Control* (Englewood Cliffs, NJ: Prentice Hall, 1991), 39.

19. Marcus Buckingham and Curt Coffman, *First, Break All the Rules* (New York: Simon & Schuster, 1999).

20. Taibi Kahler, *The Process Communication Model* (Little Rock, AR: Kahler Communications, 1982).

21. Martin Bromiley, "Have You Ever Made a Mistake?" *Bulletin of the Royal College of Anaesthetists*, no. 48 (March 2008): 2442–2445.

22. Barry Syrulaga, "Skier Lindsay Vonn Is Top U.S. Hopeful at 2010 Vancouver Olympics," *Washington Post*, February 9, 2010.

Index

Note: Page numbers followed by f or t refer to figures or tables, respectively.

Belong to the Quality Community!

Established in 1946, ASQ is a global community of quality experts in all fields and industries. ASQ is dedicated to the promotion and advancement of quality tools, principles, and practices in the workplace and in the community.

The Society also serves as an advocate for quality. Its members have informed and advised the U.S. Congress, government agencies, state legislatures, and other groups and individuals worldwide on quality-related topics.

Vision

By making quality a global priority, an organizational imperative, and a personal ethic, ASQ becomes the community of choice for everyone who seeks quality technology, concepts, or tools to improve themselves and their world.

ASQ is...

- More than 90,000 individuals and 700 companies in more than 100 countries
- The world's largest organization dedicated to promoting quality
- A community of professionals striving to bring quality to their work and their lives
- The administrator of the Malcolm Baldrige National Quality Award
- A supporter of quality in all sectors including manufacturing, service, healthcare, government, and education
- YOU

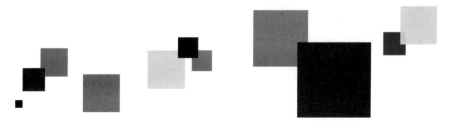

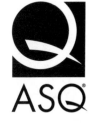

Visit www.asq.org for more information.

ASQ Membership

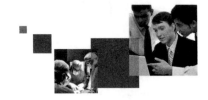

Research shows that people who join associations experience increased job satisfaction, earn more, and are generally happier*. ASQ membership can help you achieve this while providing the tools you need to be successful in your industry and to distinguish yourself from your competition. So why wouldn't you want to be a part of ASQ?

Networking

Have the opportunity to meet, communicate, and collaborate with your peers within the quality community through conferences and local ASQ section meetings, ASQ forums or divisions, ASQ Communities of Quality discussion boards, and more.

Professional Development

Access a wide variety of professional development tools such as books, training, and certifications at a discounted price. Also, ASQ certifications and the ASQ Career Center help enhance your quality knowledge and take your career to the next level.

Solutions

Find answers to all your quality problems, big and small, with ASQ's Knowledge Center, mentoring program, various e-newsletters, *Quality Progress* magazine, and industry-specific products.

Access to Information

Learn classic and current quality principles and theories in ASQ's Quality Information Center (QIC), *ASQ Weekly* e-newsletter, and product offerings.

Advocacy Programs

ASQ helps create a better community, government, and world through initiatives that include social responsibility, Washington advocacy, and Community Good Works.

Visit www.asq.org/membership for more information on ASQ membership.

*2008, The William E. Smith Institute for Association Research

ASQ Certification

ASQ certification is formal recognition by ASQ that an individual has demonstrated a proficiency within, and comprehension of, a specified body of knowledge at a point in time. Nearly 150,000 certifications have been issued. ASQ has members in more than 100 countries, in all industries, and in all cultures. ASQ certification is internationally accepted and recognized.

Benefits to the Individual

- New skills gained and proficiency upgraded
- Investment in your career
- Mark of technical excellence
- Assurance that you are current with emerging technologies
- Discriminator in the marketplace
- Certified professionals earn more than their uncertified counterparts
- Certification is endorsed by more than 125 companies

Benefits to the Organization

- Investment in the company's future
- Certified individuals can perfect and share new techniques in the workplace
- Certified staff are knowledgeable and able to assure product and service quality

Quality is a global concept. It spans borders, cultures, and languages. No matter what country your customers live in or what language they speak, they demand quality products and services. You and your organization also benefit from quality tools and practices. Acquire the knowledge to position yourself and your organization ahead of your competition.

Certifications Include

- Biomedical Auditor – CBA
- Calibration Technician – CCT
- HACCP Auditor – CHA
- Pharmaceutical GMP Professional – CPGP
- Quality Inspector – CQI
- Quality Auditor – CQA
- Quality Engineer – CQE
- Quality Improvement Associate – CQIA
- Quality Technician – CQT
- Quality Process Analyst – CQPA
- Reliability Engineer – CRE
- Six Sigma Black Belt – CSSBB
- Six Sigma Green Belt – CSSGB
- Software Quality Engineer – CSQE
- Manager of Quality/Organizational Excellence – CMQ/OE

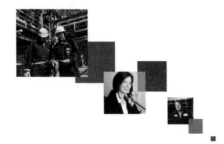

ASQ Training

Classroom-based Training

ASQ offers training in a traditional classroom setting on a variety of topics. Our instructors are quality experts and lead courses that range from one day to four weeks, in several different cities. Classroom-based training is designed to improve quality and your organization's bottom line. Benefit from quality experts; from comprehensive, cutting-edge information; and from peers eager to share their experiences.

Web-based Training

Virtual Courses

ASQ's virtual courses provide the same expert instructors, course materials, interaction with other students, and ability to earn CEUs and RUs as our classroom-based training, without the hassle and expenses of travel. Learn in the comfort of your own home or workplace. All you need is a computer with Internet access and a telephone.

Self-paced Online Programs

These online programs allow you to work at your own pace while obtaining the quality knowledge you need. Access them whenever it is convenient for you, accommodating your schedule.

Some Training Topics Include
- Auditing
- Basic Quality
- Engineering
- Education
- Healthcare
- Government
- Food Safety
- ISO
- Leadership
- Lean
- Quality Management
- Reliability
- Six Sigma
- Social Responsibility

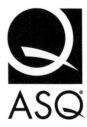

Visit www.asq.org/training for more information.